Confluences of Medicine in Medieval Japan

Confluences of Medicine in Medieval Japan

Buddhist Healing, Chinese Knowledge, Islamic Formulas, and Wounds of War

Andrew Edmund Goble

University of Hawai'i Press
Honolulu

Printed in the United States of America

17 16 15 14 13 12 11 6 5 4 3 2 1

Library of Congress Cataloging-in-Publication Data

Goble, Andrew Edmund.

Confluences of medicine in medieval Japan :
Buddhist healing, Chinese knowledge, Islamic formulas,
and wounds of war / Andrew Edmund Goble.

p. cm.

Includes bibliographical references and index.

ISBN 978-0-8248-3500-2 (cloth : alk. paper)

1. Medicine—Japan—Early works to 1800. 2. Medicine,
Chinese—Japan—Early works to 1800. 3. Kajiwara, Seizen, ca. 1265–ca. 1337.
Man'anpo. 4. Kajiwara, Seizen, ca. 1265–ca. 1337. Ton'isho. I. Title.

R624.G63 2011

610.952—dc22

2010052953

University of Hawai'i Press books are printed on acid-free
paper and meet the guidelines for permanence and
durability of the Council on Library Resources.

Designed by Janette Thompson (Jansom)

Printed by Sheridan Books, Inc.

CONTENTS

Acknowledgments ix

Introduction xiii

CHAPTER 1 The Kamakura Context 1

CHAPTER 2 Song Medicine: A View from Japan 25

CHAPTER 3 A Silk Road of Pharmaceuticals and Formulas 46

CHAPTER 4 Leprosy, Buddhist Karmic Illness, and Song Medicine 67

CHAPTER 5 Warfare, Wound Medicine, and Song Medical Knowledge 89

Epilogue: Engaging Song Medical Knowledge 113

Abbreviations 121

Notes 123

Glossary 159

Bibliography 167

Index 191

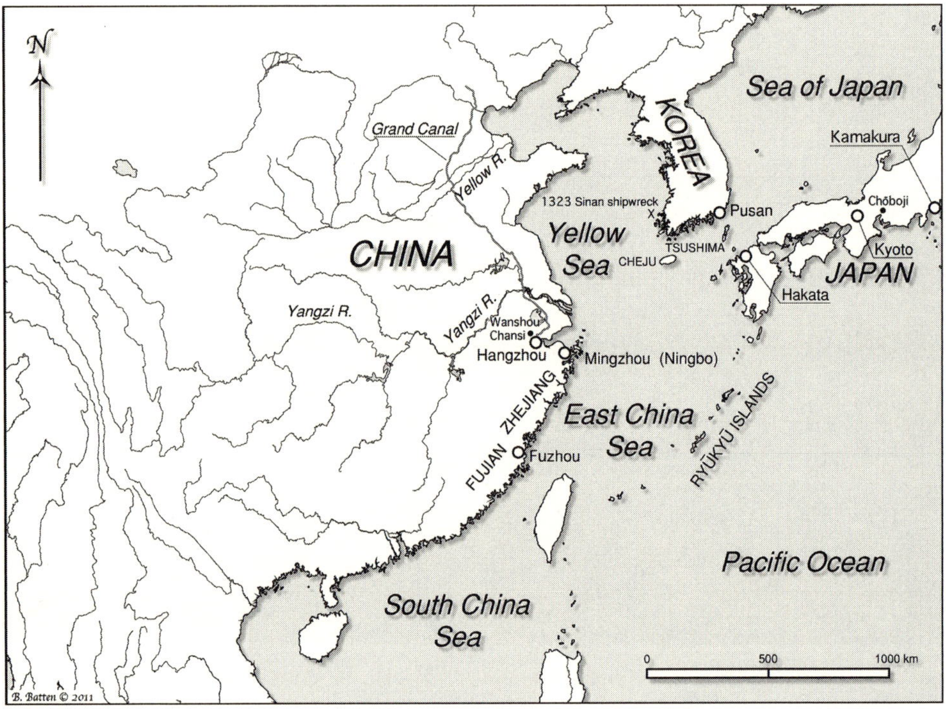

Japan in East Asia

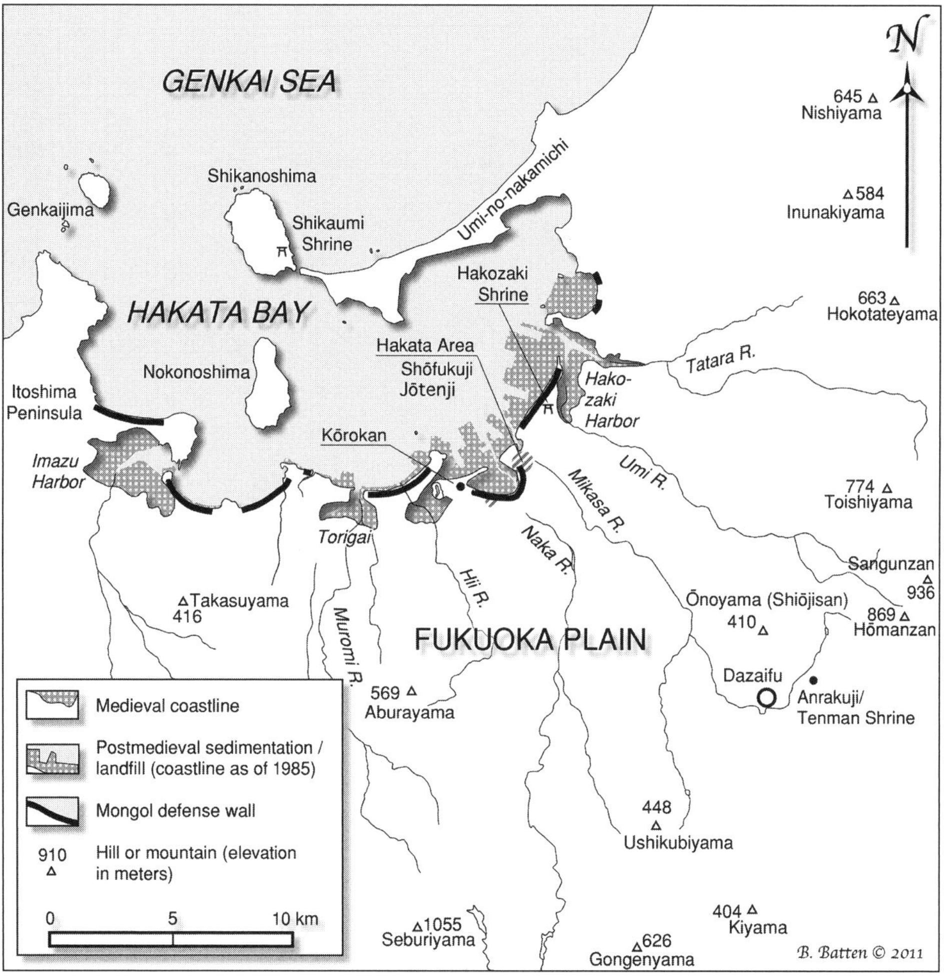
GENKAI SEA
Genkaijima
Shikanoshima
Shikaumi Shrine
Umi-no-nakamichi
HAKATA BAY
Nokonoshima
Itoshima Peninsula
Imazu Harbor
Hakozaki Shrine
Hakata Area
Shōfukuji
Jōtenji
Kōrokan
Hako-zaki Harbor
Tatara R.
Umi R.
Mikasa R.
Naka R.
Hii R.
Muromi R.
Torigai
645 Nishiyama
584 Inunakiyama
663 Hokotateyama
774 Toishiyama
Sangunzan 936
869 Hōmanzan
Ōnoyama (Shiōjisan) 410
Takasuyama 416
FUKUOKA PLAIN
569 Aburayama
Dazaifu
Anrakuji/ Tenman Shrine
448 Ushikubiyama
404 Kiyama
1055 Seburiyama
626 Gongenyama
Medieval coastline
Postmedieval sedimentation / landfill (coastline as of 1985)
Mongol defense wall
910 Hill or mountain (elevation in meters)
0 5 10 km
B. Batten © 2011

Hakata

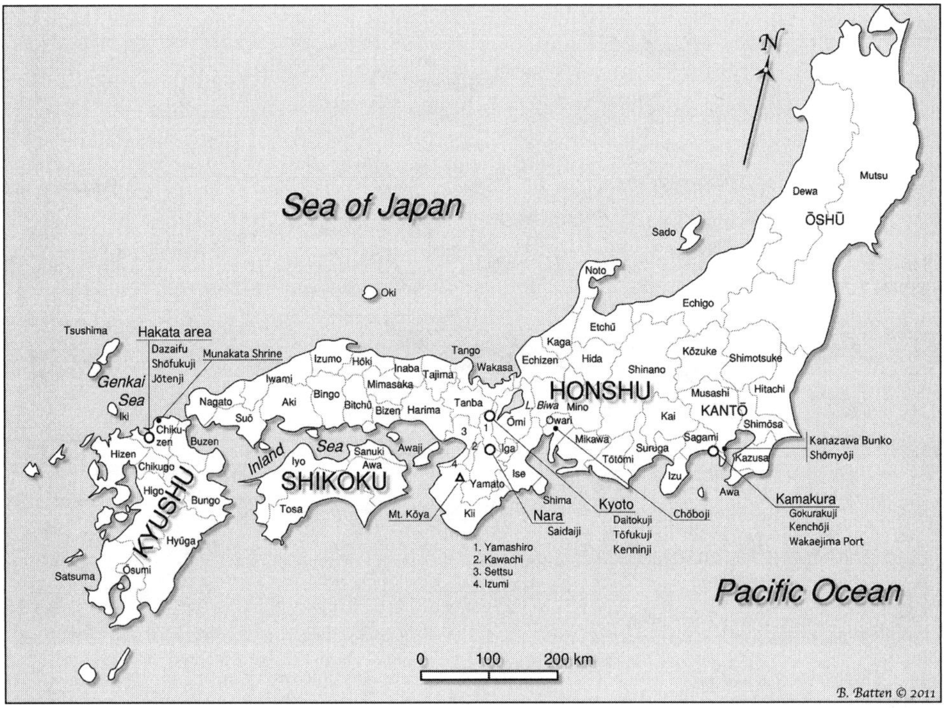

Medieval Japan

ACKNOWLEDGMENTS

The present volume is one of the results of a long-term research project on medicine in premodern Japan that I embarked upon in late 1993, supported by a generous grant from the Japan Foundation. Since that first step into a new area of research, I have been fortunate to receive support from a number of people and institutions. Without this, my window on the riches of medical history would have been far smaller.

My biggest debt of gratitude is owed to the Department of the History of Medicine of the Oriental Medicine Research Institute of the Kitasato Institute in Tokyo, and to its head, Professor Kosoto Hiroshi. In addition to facilitating my access to Chinese and Japanese medical texts, Professor Kosoto has generously provided various introductions, shared his knowledge, and fielded what must have seemed over the years endless questions about terminology, citations, interpretation, and materia medica. The department has ensured a productive research environment by allowing me unfettered access to its facilities, providing "my" desk, and has made it possible to enjoy convenient lodgings. Researchers and staff in the department have provided a wide variety of assistance. Of the many individuals, I would like to thank in particular Mayanagi Makoto (now of Ibaragi University), Machi Senjūrō (now of Nishōgakusha University), Amano Yōsuke, Tomobe Kazuhiro, Guo Xiumei, Minamizaki Kumiko, and Ōtsu Yukie. Professor Mayanagi has generously shared his expertise in Chinese medical bibliography, his knowledge of the broader field, and I have enjoyed his company at a number of international conferences; the 2010 Mito conference was especially memorable. Professor Hanawa Toshihiko, head of the Research Institute, has also provided his encouragement.

Among others who have been generous with their time and knowledge, I would like to thank Professor Sakai Shizu of Juntendo University for facilitating my initial contacts in the world of Japanese medical history;

and the late Mr. Sōda Hajime for sharing his expertise and part of his private collection. At an early stage of my research, the Historiographical Institute of the University of Tokyo provided valuable support; Professors Kuroda Hideo, Ishigami Eiichi, and Kondō Shigekazu were both professionally and personally very helpful. I am grateful also to the resources and staff of the Kyōu Shooku of Takeda Pharmaceuticals in Ōsaka, of the Naitō Kinen Kusuri Hakubutsukan in Aichi, and of the Naikaku Bunko of the National Archives of Japan in Tokyo.

Many others have provided various support, materials, opportunities to present fruits (sometimes raw) of research, or feedback. I would like to thank Bruce Batten, Alex Bay, Tom Conlan, Ed Drott, Karl Friday, Frances Garret, Bettina Gramlich-Oka, Alan Grapard, TJ Hinrichs, Ann Jannetta, Bill Johnston, Neil McMullin, Lori Meeks, Kate Nakai, Nabeshima Naoki, David Neilson, Elizabeth Oyler, David Quinter, Luke Roberts, Ken Robinson, Nathan Sivin, Mark Unno, Haruko Wakabayashi, and Duncan Williams. Bruce has also provided thoughtful counsel and furnished the maps that grace the book. I would also like to thank Yun Xia for generously providing me with her meticulous and informed proofreading on more than one occasion.

Some elements of this book (mainly in chapters 2, 3, and 5) have appeared in earlier versions in an article in the *Japanese Journal of Medical History*, an article in *Monumenta Nipponica* (*MN*), and in a chapter of the edited collection *Tools of Culture*. That material has, however, been substantially reshaped and expanded, and in the case of the *MN* article, some portions were not utilized. That is, this book represents an expansion, evolution, updating, and culmination of research rather than a reproduction of earlier material.

At the University of Hawai'i Press, I would like to thank Pat Crosby for her encouragement, various suggestions, and professionalism. The efforts of Stephanie Chun and Lee S. Motteler in the editorial and copyediting phases have also been greatly appreciated. I wish also to express my thanks to the two reviewers of the manuscript for their rigorous and extensive feedback; it has been very helpful.

At the Kyoto National Museum, I wish to express my gratitude to Director General Sasaki Jōhei and to Ms. Sakaguchi Satoko for facilitating the permission to use, and the acquisition of, the image from Kano Tanyū's *Kishitsu emaki* (held in the Museum's collection) which is used on the cover.

I will also take this opportunity to thank some people without whose support my career would have taken a very different path: my mother, Beth Perry Goble, for her belief in knowledge and education; the late Hal Bolitho for his warmth and advice on where to pursue graduate study; the late Jeff Mass for his friendship, mentoring, and scholarship; Uwayokote Masataka for welcoming an eager student and ensuring that I was equipped with my professional tools; and John Weik, my first teacher of Japanese history, for his ongoing friendship and for first sparking my interest in medical history so long ago.

Last but not least, words are inadequate to express my immense gratitude to Michiyo Horiguchi Goble, who has with great patience lived with this book as long as myself, and who has managed to keep producing her fine pottery despite the unpredictable rhythms of my research. Finally I can say, "*Tadaima.*" It is with love and appreciation that I dedicate this book to her—and in memory of Peaches.

INTRODUCTION

This book, the first monograph in English to examine aspects of medieval Japanese medical history, is largely based on a study of the medical writings of the Buddhist priest and physician Kajiwara Shōzen 梶原性全 (1265–1337).[1] His two extant works—the *Ton'ishō* 頓医抄 (Book of the Simple Physician) of 1304[2] and the *Man'anpō* 万安方 (Myriad Relief Prescriptions) of 1327[3]—are landmarks in Japanese medical history. The former is the first medical work written in Japanese rather than in Chinese script and the first medical work that was intended for wide dissemination. The latter, written in Chinese and directed at a more learned audience, is the most extensive medical compilation produced in Japan prior to at least the seventeenth century. It is longer than the much better-known tenth-century (984) compilation the *Ishinpō* 医心方 (Formulas from the Heart of Medicine),[4] which is based on hand-written Chinese medical texts produced no later than the eighth century. Both *Ton'ishō* and *Man'anpō* draw extensively on Chinese printed medical works of the Song (and Yuan) era, and at the very minimum they represent the first substantial updating of Japanese understanding of Chinese medical knowledge in over three centuries. Those three centuries witnessed significant developments in Chinese medicine. Surprisingly, however, Shōzen's writings have not been extensively studied. The present work is the first in any language to focus on them.

The theme of this book is the dissemination and appropriation of Song medical knowledge in thirteenth- and fourteenth-century Japan. That process was part of the second wave of Chinese cultural influence in Japanese history (which is perhaps most commonly associated with the implantation of Chan or Zen Buddhism). Accordingly, we will be looking at Japanese medical history in the context of contact and interaction in East Asia. Concomitantly, we will be looking at Chinese medical knowledge in a wider East Asian context rather than solely in the context of medical history in China. In doing so, I both recognize the contemporary existence of an East Asian macroculture, of which medicine was an integral component, and build upon recent scholarly trends in the study of medieval Japan. These trends see medieval history as naturally incorporating contacts in East Asia rather than as a process that somehow stops at the low-tide mark of the Japanese islands, and they see overseas contacts as continuous rather than sporadic.[5]

In looking at the impact of Song medical knowledge, I also hope to provide some sense of how that was shaped, facilitated, or limited. After all, knowledge is transmitted in historical context and by human beings rather than through some amorphous or inevitable process. Chapters 2 through 5 are devoted to different topics on medicine and medical knowledge, and in those chapters various factors and contingencies that are germane to those topics will emerge naturally. However, I have devoted chapter 1 to an exploration of some broader elements that will help us address the basic question of what made it possible for Kajiwara Shōzen to gain access to Song medical knowledge and to write his landmark texts.

Chapter 1, "The Kamakura Context," draws attention to four salient factors. First, I note the fact that Japan's aristocratic political elite in central Japan had very little contact with the outside world and very little interest in exploring new knowledge. In contrast, people living in northwestern Kyushu (the southern island lying roughly halfway between central Japan and southern Chinese ports) had increasingly greater contact and a much more expansive worldview. One manifestation of this was the growth of a Chinese merchant community around Hakata Bay and the development of international contacts beyond the narrow purview of the central polity. Second, while there was very little official Japanese cultural interaction with China after the 850s, I draw attention to the growth, after the 1150s, of contacts with China in which the role of Buddhist priests was central. That interaction utilized links with the Chinese merchant community, but it drew more fundamentally upon what appear to have been long-term Buddhist networks in East Asia. These networks, while to date not given the attention they deserve by scholars, operated through a combination of institutional linkages and personal acquaintances that provided a web of contacts through which information could be shared. The third factor I note is the growth of Buddhist charitable activity in Japan during the thirteenth century, most notably that associated with the newly formed

Ritsu Precept sect of Buddhism. This sect was devoted to the cult of the Mañjuśrī Buddha and placed great emphasis on attending to the spiritual and physical needs of the bereft in society. From the mid-1200s, the sect received official patronage from Japan's new warrior government in the eastern city of Kamakura and founded what soon became the largest medical facility in premodern Japanese history. Kajiwara Shōzen was a Ritsu Precept sect priest and worked at that facility. The fourth factor I note is the expansive attitude towards China and Chinese that we find in the Kamakura warrior government and more generally among the population of Kamakura, which by the mid-1200s was Japan's second-largest city. Trade with China was actively encouraged, and Kamakura developed new sea routes that connected it to the East Asian maritime networks. Chinese goods were prized, and printed Song books were eagerly acquired. In Kajiwara Shōzen's time, Kamakura provided a unique environment that facilitated the engagement of Song medical knowledge.

In exploring the appropriation and dissemination of Song medical knowledge in chapters 2 through 5, I look at two general themes and at two topics in each of those themes. The first theme that I take up is the availability and shape of Song medical knowledge, and the two topics are the availability and influence of written medical texts and of materia medica. The second theme that I take up is the impact of Song medical knowledge on medical issues of great concern in contemporary Japanese society. I look first at the problem of leprosy 癩 and second at the issue of battle injury. Throughout, readers will be able to observe the interplay between existing and new understandings of medicine and medicines; the mechanics of the appropriation and incorporation of new information; and some of the interaction of knowledge and perspectives drawn from three broader medical systems: the Japanese, the Chinese, and the Buddhist. I hasten to add that these medical systems were not exclusive nor unchanging, and they present challenges to precise definition. However, they were contemporaneously recognized as components of medicine in Japan.

Chapter 2, "Song Medicine: A View from Japan," focuses on the understanding of Song medicine that Kajiwara Shōzen was able to gain from printed Song medical works. Against a background of the scarcity of Japanese medical works and the plethora of information that became available in a new media as a result of the Song printing revolution, I first sketch the contours of what is best understood as the appropriating context of Song medicine. The chapter examines the variety of Song printed medical works and then looks in more detail at some of the works that Shōzen consulted. From this, readers can gain a sense of what he would have understood of Song medicine and how Song medicine would have shaped his idea of medicine. The chapter then looks at how Shōzen benefited from Song knowledge, both in terms of learning new things and in terms of identifying shortcomings in Japanese medicine. Considered are a number of general examples and then some that relate to women's medicine.

In chapter 3, "A Silk Road of Pharmaceuticals and Formulas," I focus on the materia medica and formulas that appear in Song medical texts. I note how some changes in the Chinese pharmaceutical regime from the Tang through the Song—and an extensive trade network that brought materia medica to Japan from as far away as the Middle East—combined to reshape the form and content of medicines in medieval Japan. The early portions of the chapter explore technical matters in some detail. I do so in order to provide information on the variety of materia medica; to emphasize the fact that the natural world is integral to medical history; and to convey a sense of the significant technical challenges involved in introducing new formulas, new weights and measures, and new materia medica into Japanese medicine. It is perhaps fair to say that the topics of technology, science, and technical translation during the medieval period have not been well studied to date, and it is hoped that this will serve to shed some light on them. Readers will also discover that aspects of Islamic medicine that had been incorporated into Chinese medicine were also conveyed to medieval Japan. To illustrate the rich complexity that underlies this, I describe how Shōzen was able to understand a new Song category of illness—Disorders of Qi—in the treatment of which Islamic-influenced formulas were prominent, because it resonated with understandings of Buddhist disease etiology with which he was already familiar.

In chapters 4 and 5, the focus shifts to an examination of two medical issues that were of contemporary concern. In taking up the topics of leprosy and battle injury, it is possible to explore how and why Song knowledge was applied in two quite different areas of medicine. We see that the impact of Song knowledge was varied.

Chapter 4, "Leprosy, Buddhist Karmic Illness, and Song Medicine," takes up one of the most socially, religiously, and medically complex afflictions of the medieval era. Whereas prior scholarship has given much attention to leprosy as a social and religious matter—examining issues of discrimination and marginalization and aspects of Buddhist teachings, particularly the notion of karma, that may have justified some discrimination—in taking it up as a medical matter, we not only gain insight into changes in medicine, we are also able to appreciate that it was a more nuanced phenomenon than generally represented. I also provide the first detailed description of this affliction. The chapter starts with a look at leprosy as a clinical matter and notes the symptoms and the treatments available. I then move to Shōzen's initial understanding of the Buddhist etiology of leprosy as a karmic disease. While the concept is well known, there is little understanding of what this meant as a medical matter in medieval Japan, and so I then explore that issue. It is apparent that the idea of karmic illness was not well understood and that the idea of leprosy as a karmic illness was not fixed. One major discovery is that, as a result of clinical experience and acquaintance with Song medicine, Shōzen came to reject the idea of leprosy as a Buddhist karmic illness. This provides a clear example of how existing understanding of an illness that was not based on medical knowledge could be reevaluated in light of clinical experience and new Song knowledge.

Chapter 5, "Warfare, Wound Medicine, and Song Medical Knowledge," pursues the medical response to the unprecedented explosion of violence and warfare in the early fourteenth century. This topic permits us to explore a different range of factors that shaped the availability and reception of Song medical knowledge, and it identifies an area where Song medical knowledge was not obviously more advanced than Japanese medical knowledge. Wound medicine is of great interest because it was not a recognized area of medical specialty prior to the fourteenth century, despite the long-term existence of the Japanese warrior class: It became so in direct response to a pressing need. Kajiwara Shōzen dealt with the topic only in passing, and, since he died in 1337 after the completion of the *Man'anpō* in 1327 and soon after the destruction of Kamakura in 1333, we of course do not know how he might have responded to the new medical need. But we are able to learn how other physicians responded by examining the first texts written on wound medicine. We learn that physicians extrapolated from existing medical knowledge found in popular medicine (which includes information of the type noted in the *Ton'ishō*) rather than from Chinese textual knowledge. The exigencies of the times and the level of literacy of physicians may have been factors in this. It is also clear, however, that knowledge of wound treatment found in Chinese books likely to have been available in Japan would not have been particularly helpful. Despite this,

I identify two ways in which Song medicine influenced Japanese wound medicine. The first was that some materia medica acquired through overseas trade and utilized because of the introduction of Song formulas was integral to wound medicine. The second influence was that the conceptual basis for the field of wound medicine was derived from Song medical writing.

I conclude this study with some thoughts on what we are able to learn of the processes by which knowledge was acquired, understood, and appropriated in the premodern era. In addition, I suggest that the rich detail made available in Shōzen's work at least suggests something of the manner of scientific inquiry in premodern Japan.

Since I will be drawing on Shōzen's two writings to learn about the influence of Song medicine in Japan and will not be focusing simply on these works, a brief overview of the structure and content of the *Ton'ishō* and *Man'anpō* at this point will be useful.[6]

The *Ton'ishō* is written in Japanese, which is to say it combines Chinese characters and Japanese katakana phonetic syllabary in Japanese word order. Though there are occasional passages in Chinese (and a chapter titled "Secret Transmissions of Medicines" is in Chinese), citations from Chinese works are almost always translated into Japanese, and Shōzen's own comments are written primarily in colloquial Japanese. His reason for doing so was twofold. On the one hand, he felt that Japanese physicians did not have high levels of literacy and rarely consulted medical works. On the other hand, he felt that medical knowledge should be made available rather than not shared.

> When I looked at a certain medical work [it was evident that] this matter [treatment for diarrhea] was an exceedingly important one. There is a major oral transmission, and even though it is a secret matter, my aim in writing in phonetic syllabary is to make things widely known to people and to help everyone in the realm. The average physician either focuses on profit and conceals things which are not difficult, or else out of self-interest keeps secret those things which are of benefit. This is absolutely contrary to the heart of heaven and in no way benefits people's bodies. As to secret matters, from the very beginning I have encountered them in explanations of teachers, in oral traditions, and also in [over] thirty books; and in my heart I believed that this was wrong. Having come to this understanding, I have used it as my strong guide when treating. This alone is the core of this path of medicine.[7]

The text used in the modern facsimile edition of the *Ton'ishō* is roughly 3,000 leaves (pages) in length. A separate handwritten copy that I also used is roughly 2,700 leaves in length. *Ton'ishō* contains a little over 1,400 formulas, cites around fifty-five Chinese medical works, and is divided into fifty chapters. The chapters are not based on a single organizing principle but on such things as etiology, specific medical challenge, symptoms, or topics of interest. While being aware that not all ailments noted in premodern East Asian medicine have exact correlations with modern medical understandings—and there is always the positivist danger of anachronistically trying to identify something—I will describe the chapters as covering the following topics: Cold and heat affecting five viscera and six bowels; wind ailments; cold damage disorders (exogenous febrile disease); abdominal mass (lump); corpse transmitted disease; ailments of the qi; vomiting and sunstroke; hemorrhoids, abdominal edema, and swelling; consumption 虚損 and lumbago; various urological problems; asthmatic and esophageal problems; depression and madness; ear, nose, and throat; oral cavity and mouth; colic and testicular problems; diabetes; bleedings from bodily cavities; noxious factors (which can cause mental imbalance) and stroke; sores and carbuncles; seven chapters on women's medicine (menstruation, miscellaneous ailments, conception, pregnancy, birth, postpartum); leprosy; five chapters on pediatrics; permitted and prohibited foods; pulse diagnosis; acupuncture and moxibustion; viscera; sexual intercourse; ethos of the physician; characteristics of medicines and flavors; secret transmissions on medicines; and nurturing longevity.

The *Man'anpō* is written in Chinese, suggesting that the intended audience was educated medical professionals (initially perhaps those in Shōzen's lineage), Buddhist priests, and the better-educated members of the social elite. Shōzen's comments are also in Chinese. One also finds, however, that Japanese pronunciations (in katakana phonetic syllabary) for names of materia medica and ailments are often provided alongside the Chinese terms.

The *Man'anpō* in the modern facsimile printed edition is roughly 6,800 leaves in length. It cites at least 270 Chinese medical works (there are also some three Japanese medical works mentioned), although not all are direct citations. It contains over 3,100 formulas. The version completed in 1327 was transcribed by Shōzen with the assistance of his son Fuyukage, an émigré Chinese by the name of Daoguang, and another anonymous Chinese. It consists of fifty chapters. After Shōzen's death, other of his writings were added to give us the extant *Man'anpō* of sixty-two chapters (plus a detailed table of contents). We may consider this his magnum opus.

In the *Man'anpō,* as with the *Ton'ishō,* while in general each chapter has an introduction and we find throughout comments of varying length by Shōzen, formulas and instructions for preparation comprise the bulk of each chapter. The chapters cover such topics as endogenous wind syndrome/apoplexy; head colds; bad skin and various wind afflictions; cold damage; sunstroke; malaria; choleric disease; chest pain; disorders of qi; consumption 虚労; phlegm retention syndrome; edema; colic; jaundice; diarrhea; leukorrhea; bowel and urinary problems; sores and carbuncles; various swellings; incised wounds; *kakke* 脚気 (beriberi, articular rheumatism, gout); scrotal and testicular problems; piles and hemorrhoids; eyes, ears, and nose; and oral cavity and throat. There are eight chapters on obstetrics, which are devoted to the topics of pregnancy, wind syndrome during pregnancy, prescriptions for calming the fetus, characteristics at different ages of pregnancy and charts for tranquil births, eighteen prepartum indications, twenty-one postpartum ailments, and postpartum consumption. There are eleven chapters on pediatrics that cover such things as cutting the umbilical cord, insufficient milk being produced by the mother, fright, wind syndrome, coughing and dyspnea, night sweats, various infant malnutrition ailments, vomiting and diarrhea, and miscellaneous ailments. The twelve chapters later added to the original fifty cover such topics as theory of medicine, viscera and anatomy, points ("holes") for moxibustion, a two-volume referential identification guide to Chinese and Japanese names for materia medica, and a two-volume guide to tastes and flavors of medicines.

This study will touch on only a portion of the material contained in the *Ton'ishō* and the *Man'anpō.* It by no means exhausts the range of topics that may be engaged, but it is hoped that this initial exploration may suggest other areas that invite inquiry. I also hope that it will convey some sense that medical texts can tell us much about such issues as medicine and society or the appropriation and construction of knowledge, as well as making the obvious point that it is intrinsically worthwhile learning about medicine and medicines.

Chapter 1

THE KAMAKURA CONTEXT

Coinciding with the onset of a second wave of Chinese cultural influence on Japan, the Kamakura era was characterized by unprecedented change and mobility, new opportunities for interaction, and challenges to existing forms of institutional, religious, and cultural authority.[1] While this did not mean that older forms and conventions were suddenly swept aside or even that changes proceeded completely or uniformly, the larger picture is clear.

Three broad developments are particularly noteworthy. First was the establishment of Japan's first warrior government, the Kamakura *bakufu,* and more generally the attendant political and cultural rise of the warrior class at the ultimate expense of the old imperial aristocracy. Second, in the religious realm, a variety of teachings bypassed the traditional monastic establishment and reached new audiences. Teachings and sects that focused on issues of salvation and psychological support in the present life, such as the Pure Land, Lotus, and Ritsu Precept sects, made extensive efforts to address the spiritual and existential needs of the commoner population. Song-style Zen (Chan) monastic Buddhism, catalyzed from the mid-1200s by warrior patronage of Chinese monks, facilitated the transfer and appropriation of a new range of cultural and intellectual understandings. Third, the adoption and appropriation of elements of Song Chinese culture were facilitated by active human and commercial engagement with China and the broader East Asian maritime trade network. Channeled particularly through the cosmopolitan port cities of Ningbo in south China and Hakata in Kyushu, these contacts created new routes for the acquisition and dissemination of information.

In order to appreciate how these different elements created an environment conducive to the exploration of Song medical knowledge, I will briefly survey the following topics. First, to get some sense of the background to the new wave of knowledge, I consider the difference in attitudes to the outside world between Japan's aristocratic elite in the city of Kyoto in central Japan and nonaristocrats near Hakata Bay on the southern island of Kyushu. Next I will shed some light on the Buddhist networks that facilitated cultural and intellectual contacts. Finally, in order to get a sense of Kajiwara Shōzen's working context, I look first at the Ritsu Precept sect and medical facilities in Kamakura and then at some aspects of the cosmopolitan milieu of that city.

THE OUTSIDE WORLD VIEWED FROM KYOTO AND KYUSHU

The traditional view of Japanese engagement of Chinese knowledge and interactions with Chinese people between the early 600s and the late twelfth century identifies two general phases. First, from the early 600s through the mid-800s (coinciding with the dispatch of diplomatic missions to China in the Prince Shōtoku, Nara, and early-Heian eras), Japan's political elite actively pursued formal diplomatic relations, eagerly acquired the fruits of Chinese civilization, and built what we call classical Japanese civilization. Second, from the mid-800s (coinciding with the mid- through late-Heian eras), due to a combination of a cultural self-confidence, the political turmoil into which Tang China descended, and restriction on overseas contact imposed by the Northern Song government after it was established in the 960s, a sedentary hereditary aristocracy located in the imperial capital of Heian (Kyoto) lost interest in this outside world and turned inward.

While this provides a useful overview of the engagement with the outside world of the aristocratic ruling elite in central Japan, it does not tell the full story. Once one moves outside the center and takes account of activity in areas considered peripheral by the center, one gets a different sense of both "Japan" and of the rhythms of engagement with the outside world (meaning, here, China). Northwestern Kyushu, which was oriented to the sea as much as it was to the landed interior of the Japanese islands, is particularly important to this reorientation. An understanding of northwestern Kyushu helps us to appreciate the epistemological circumscription of the Heian elite and also some mechanisms by which that was circumvented from the late 1100s. Let us then look in turn at the worldview of the Heian elite and the dynamics of northwestern Kyushu.

As is well known, contact with China from the early 600s enabled Japanese civilization to make a qualitative leap forward. One substantial legacy of this was the creation of a biliterate elite culture in which works were written in Chinese 漢文 as well as in Japanese 和文. The two orthographies were considered complementary rather than adversarial, in a manner analogous to the roles of Shinto and Buddhism in the religious sphere. Thus, while the literary masterpieces written in Japanese are frequently privileged as defining classical Japanese literature, it is important to recognize that works written in Chinese (laws, judicial decisions, official documents, medical works, chronicles, diaries, philosophical writings, poetry, Buddhist writings) are equally part of the written product of the Japanese past. In fact, the bulk of the premodern written corpus is in Chinese.

Another result of the China contact was that by the tenth century the Heian aristocracy had constructed a Japanese tradition of Chinese classical learning that was largely based upon Tang Chinese materials produced prior to the mid-ninth century. While this focus is understandable enough in terms of time frame, other factors served to reinforce it. One factor was that few educated Heian era Japanese (and as far as we can tell, no member of the aristocracy) went abroad after the 850s, and thus there was minimal opportunity to acquire texts and send them back. Another factor may have been the general chaos attending the decline of the Tang, during which few new works were produced and many physical copies of existing material were destroyed. Finally, the Northern Song government restricted the export of Chinese works, which meant a virtual interdiction on such things as the printed encyclopedias and major medical works whose compilation the Northern Song had sponsored. But an equally important reason for lack of interest in post-Tang materials, even when they were acquirable, lay in some social forces and attitudes to knowledge internal to the Heian aristocracy.

Aristocratic families maintained distinction through their cultural capital. Thus, for example, experts in law or the Confucian classics achieved such status because they hereditarily monopolized textual interpretations and conventions of reading. They also guarded closely, as private family treasures, the handwritten scrolls on which texts were written. Thus, as Ivo Smits has shown in his study of the book collections of two important twelfth-century political figures, book (or scroll) collecting and ownership of a collection had major ramifications. A well-placed collector was able to use the intertwined social and political dynamics of the patronage and network building around which aristocratic society functioned to shape intellectual endeavor and to prescribe a certain body of material as the canon. Thus, when from the mid-1100s Chinese printed books, a revolutionary new media, began to become available from Southern Song traders, the works in demand were by and large new editions of known and valued materials. There was little interest among aristocrats in exploring the works of contemporary Song authors, who were in the process of creating a new Chinese written corpus and rethinking their classical tradition. In addition, financial considerations may have come into play. Only the wealthier aristocrats—those already at the top of the social hierarchy—may have been able to afford them. Even in the 1260s, a full set of the *Taiping yulan* 太平御覧 encyclopedia cost about the same as a modest mansion.[2] In other words, since unfamiliar material might be a threat to existing privilege and might also require a new intellectual framework, it made little social or financial sense to acquire new knowledge.

Compounding this inner turn that oriented the aristocracy to its life in the imperial capital was the structure of domestic government, which in essence recognized local autonomy and delegated provincial administration through a hierarchy of patron-client relations. The very success of this central-local division of labor confirmed that aristocrats belonged at the center and compounded the reticence to move beyond the physical and psychological boundaries of the capital. Thus, while reports and complaints might describe some local conditions, provincial clients who traveled to the capital might contribute some firsthand descriptions, some tale literature might provide accounts of provincial doings, and property documents inscribed their own cartographic order on the world, the aristocracy's collective images of the world beyond Kyoto were mediated and imagined rather than based upon direct experience.

The desire to keep the domestic world at a mediated distance was replicated in arrangements for dealing with the overseas world, which was channeled through the government headquarters of Dazaifu 大宰府.[3] In the Kyoto mind, Dazaifu was a periphery on the edge of civilization, and for aristocrats an appointment in Dazaifu was often seen as a de facto sentence of exile. The attitude to visitors from overseas was that they had little legitimate reason to further penetrate Japanese civilization. Trade with other coastal sites might be condoned, and the Kyoto elite prized the luxury goods that foreign trade made available, but travel by foreigners to

Kyoto was rarely permitted. Moreover, while we have no way of knowing the extent of the interaction between fisherfolk or private traders on the coasts of western Japan, the Korean peninsula, or the islands between them, the officially recorded number of people and goods involved in trade was very small. All in all, as Bruce Batten has convincingly argued, Japan was a remarkably isolated country.[4]

Nonetheless, Dazaifu was responsible for enforcing the regulations governing the frequency with which and in what numbers Chinese trade ships might be granted official permission to engage in commercial activities. Any problems that arose—irregularities in ship numbers or frequency of arrival, overstaying, commercial disputes, and suchlike—were referred to Kyoto for higher action. The bureaucratic process was lengthy and thorough and seems to reflect the limited amount of trade and interaction. That is, the top-heavy arrangements were not designed for rapid responses to frequent occurrences but to confirm Kyoto's ultimate authority.

The interdiction policy was successful. Prior to the thirteenth century, references to physical interaction between aristocrats and Chinese are sparse but instructive. In 1014 the imperial court invited the Great Song priest-physician Huiqing, who was residing in Dazaifu, to provide medicine for treating eye illness. Aristocrats, however, were concerned that the medicine did not have a name, so after subjecting the issue to divination—whether the medicine was effective seems not to have been the issue—they determined that they should stop administering it.[5] In 1170, when the military aristocrat Taira Kiyomori invited the retired emperor Go-Shirakawa to visit his estate-cum-port of Fukuhara (near modern Kobe) for the specific purpose of seeing some actual Chinese visitors, one diarist remarked that "not many Chinese have come to the Court since the Engi era [901–923]."[6] In another example, in 1179 when Kiyomori suggested that a Chinese physician treat his ailing son, the son refused on the grounds that it was an insult to be treated by a foreign rather than a Japanese physician.[7]

In sum, while the information from the 1170s suggests that newer attitudes may have been emerging, there is little doubt that for a period of centuries the worldview of the Kyoto aristocracy was circumscribed. Their attitude to knowledge and the new was passive and sedentary. However, the aristocracy seems not to have felt disadvantaged by this. On the contrary, restrictions reinforced existing privileges, whether over defining a corpus of knowledge or maintaining broader political and legal authority (as has recently been suggested with respect to the issue of importing coinage).[8]

When we shift our focus, however, from Kyoto's view of foreigners and Dazaifu's role in national administration to what people seem to have been doing in the area around Dazaifu, our picture is different. Northwestern Kyushu was open to the outside world, whereas Kyoto was not. This of course was literally true, since the Dazaifu headquarters was charged with monitoring the movement of goods and people to and from overseas. But it is apparent that over time, northwestern Kyushu, located close to the Korean peninsula and halfway between Kyoto and the port cities of southern China, became oriented as much to the Asian mainland as it was to the political center of Kyoto.

By the mid-twelfth century, northwestern Kyushu had started to become an important and relatively cosmopolitan hub for private trade in maritime East Asia and a center for overlapping trade, patronage, and cultural and religious networks that operated independently of the Kyoto world. The example of the physician Huiqing noted above suggests that at least some Chinese lived in the Dazaifu area from the early eleventh century, though for what length of time and in what numbers is uncertain. By the early 1100s, however, trading activity had become sufficiently frequent (and no doubt lucrative) that Chinese merchants had established a permanent trading and warehousing site on the shore of Hakata Bay. Situated on an uninhabited and uncultivated island between two rivers that flowed into Hakata Bay, in time it became the core of the medieval port city of Hakata.

The Chinese community that appears in sources was varied. Some, like the Fujian native Zhang Guang'an, who erected a monument to his deceased parents in Ningbo, were Hakata residents but retained deep emotional ties to China.[9] Others, like the boat captain Su, married into the Japanese community and produced offspring.[10] Yet others, like Yang Rong, were born in Hakata and for business purposes could be seen as either Japanese or Chinese.[11] And women were as much a part of the community as men. In one striking example from the early 1200s, two Chinese women, a Ms. Wang and a Ms. Zhang, apparently daughters of Hakata Chinese merchants, married into the priestly family of Munakata Shrine 宗像神社. Munakata was one of the oldest and most prestigious religious institutions in western Japan, had goddesses of the sea as its tutelary deities, and was heavily involved in overseas trade. Ms. Wang and Ms. Zhang were thus insiders in three communities: Chinese, Japanese, and their own bridging one. Their offspring succeeded to headship of the shrine, they owned property in their own names, enjoyed the same access to the legal system as anybody else, and in Ms. Zhang's case, suffered as a mother.[12]

The Chinese community—ethnic Chinese, their partners, and their offspring—managed the overseas trade network that connected Hakata to south China. In the absence of adequate Japanese marine technology, it also provided the seagoing vessels that were essential for the trade. We may also assume that it provided the required linguistic skills for international trade. The broader Hakata community—which included landholders around Hakata Bay, Japanese religious institutions, and, particularly after the establishment of the Kamakura *bakufu* in 1185, members of the warrior class—also facilitated the movement of people between Japan and China. It was also receptive to Song culture and was an important node in the Buddhist networks that disseminated that culture to Japan.

BUDDHIST NETWORKS AND CHINESE MEDICINE

Scholars of interactions between Japan and East Asia, perhaps because of a long-standing bias towards official contacts and state-centered history, have overlooked one of the most important elements in understanding the flow of information and knowledge across the East China Sea: Buddhist religious networks. To be sure, the crucial role of Zen monks in diplomatic and other interactions from the thirteenth century, the wide-ranging contacts in the Japanese Buddhist world, and the movement of individual figures from institution to institution or teacher to teacher are well known. But scholars have been slow to note that Buddhist monks and their institutions made up a transnational, nonstate network that operated irrespective of the sporadic government-to-government contacts that passed for diplomacy throughout East Asia.

Almost all of the small number of Japanese who are recorded as visiting China between the 830s and the 1150s were Buddhist monks, of whom the best known are Ennin (793–864) and Jōjin 1011–1081).[13] From the 1160s, the number of monks traveling to China increased gradually. After the mid-1200s it became a steady stream, and from that time we note an equally steady flow of Chinese Zen monks to Japan. What specifically prompted this new wave of Japanese monk travelers in the mid-1100s is not entirely clear. Religious interest certainly would have played a part, since the lineages of Buddhist monks traced back to China. Greater opportunity, such as an increased frequency of shipping from Hakata or the possibility that Chinese merchants might provide introductions to Chinese teachers and institutions, may also have been a factor. And we should not forget that the Southern Song encouraged a more open engagement with the external maritime world than did the Northern Song. While perhaps no more than a few hundred Japanese made this journey prior to the fourteenth century, they had a cultural impact out of all proportion to their numbers. Following are two examples of people whose activity contributed to the dissemination of medical knowledge.

Myōan Eisai 明庵栄西 (1141–1215) was one of the first of the new wave of Buddhist travelers. Unusually, he made two trips to China, first in 1168 and then again from 1187 to 1191. In 1187 he had originally intended to make a pilgrimage to the home of Buddhism in India, but after being denied permission to transit China he decided to stay and study Zen. Under the tutelage of a highly regarded Chinese Zen master, he was recognized as having achieved enlightenment and returned to Japan as a credentialed member of a flourishing Chinese Buddhist sect. He spent the first four years after his return in the Hakata area, where, with the financial support of Chinese merchants, he took over or established several temples (the most well known being Shōfukuji 聖福寺). These were the first temples in Japan to highlight Zen practice. They were undoubtedly a religious and cultural focus for the Chinese community, part of a network of business and religious patronage, and provided Eisai with a foundation without which his efforts to introduce the new Zen teachings would have been far less successful. Eisai later sought support from the new warrior government in Kamakura as well as figures in Kyoto. By 1200 he had become established at Kenninji Temple 建仁寺 in Kyoto. Eisai's overall contribution to Zen culture and his corpus of writings need not detain us here, but it is worth noting his essay *Kissa yōjōki* 喫茶養生記 (On Drinking Tea as a Means to Long Life).[14]

The *Kissa Yōjōki* is most commonly known as a work that introduced the custom of drinking powdered green tea and thus laid the basis for a broader cultural aesthetic that has become an integral part of Japanese tradition. However, this future was not known to Eisai. His purpose in writing the *Kissa yōjōki* was to provide new information for nourishing the body and treating some specific ailments. In the introduction, he notes that tea is a Transcendent's Medicine for nurturing life 茶者養生之仙薬也; that in this age of Buddhist decline, three thousand years after the Divine Husbandman Shennong 神農 and two thousand years since the Indian healer Jīvaka 耆婆, no one can really heal, and acupuncture, moxibustion, and hotspring therapy are ineffectively applied. But since he is aware of aware of the currents of the Great Country (China), he is able to indicate some modern healing methods 近代治方. The first part of the work discusses tea, noting such things as its contribution to the harmonious functioning of the five viscera, its long tradition in India and China, and places in China associated with it. The section ends by quoting Chinese physicians to the effect that "In the case of people who do not drink tea, medicines lose their efficacy, and their illnesses cannot be treated, since their heart is weak." Eisai does not provide examples of how tea might be used, but a source from 1214 dated just one month after the foreword to the *Kissa yōjōki* records that while visiting Kamakura, Eisai prescribed tea to cure a hangover of the shogun Minamoto Sanetomo (1192–1219). Eisai also presented Sanetomo with a one-volume text that praised tea, which may have been the *Kissa yōjōki*.[15]

The second part of *Kissa yōjōki* has nothing to do with tea. It focuses on illness and medicine. Eisai lists formulas for five medical problems: what we know to be diabetes 飲水病, palsy 中風病, not-eating illness 不食病, sores 瘡病, and the ambulatory affliction of *kakke* 脚気. He discusses the provenance and preparation of Korean ginseng (good for myriad ailments) and a Five Fragrances Infusion 五香煎 whose ingredients were birthwort, aloes, musk, cloves, and frankincense. There is also a lengthy discussion of the medicinal benefits of mulberry, the oral tradition for which was conveyed to him by a Chinese physician.[16] Eisai also notes in passing that he had gained some information from an unidentified, newly arrived medical work.

The *Kissa yōjōki* thus provides our first important information on the Kamakura period engagement of Chinese medicine. Subsequent to the mention of Huiqing in 1014—and allowing that the Kyushu monk physicians who were invited to Kyoto in 1177 may have had some contact with Chinese informants—the *Kissa yōjōki* is otherwise the first evidence in nearly three centuries that knowledge of Chinese medicine was being obtained directly from living Chinese.[17] We also learn that Song medical texts were now being imported into Japan. We learn, too, that there were some health problems for which Chinese formulas from oral sources were recommended; it is implicit that they were more effective than Japanese formulas—and perhaps even that Japanese ones were inferior. But perhaps because *Kissa yōjōki* drew on such works as the Northern Song *Taiping yulan,* there are some anachronisms. For example, Eisai noted that Korean ginseng came from Song Chinese territory, which had not been the case since 1127 at the latest. Still, *Kissa yōjōki* intimates a new psychological proximity to China and hints at a broader framework within which medical knowledge might be obtained.

The second and more extended example takes as a common point the monk Enni Ben'en 円爾弁円 (1202–1280) and highlights the multistranded network of connections involved in the dissemination of Song knowledge to and within Japan. In 1235, after a dispute at his temple in Kyoto, Enni went to Hakata determined to travel to China. In Hakata he received the support of Xie Guoming 謝国明, a native of Huangzhou Province who was married to a Japanese woman and was one of the most successful Hakata Chinese merchants of the thirteenth century. His holdings included land acquired from Munakata Shrine, and he was a patron of religious institutions in both China and Japan. Leaving Hakata (no doubt with passage on a ship arranged by Guoming), Enni then spent seven years at Zhejiang Province's Wanshou Chansi 万壽禅寺 Zen temple, which in time became a prized destination for many Japanese monks and the departure point to Japan of many Chinese monks. In 1241, his training complete, Enni departed China and after an eventful voyage, which included surviving a shipwreck (two accompanying ships were lost completely) and making a forced detour through Korea, he arrived in Hakata. There he once again received support from Xie Guoming and also from the warrior Shōni Sukeyoshi (1198–1281), the head of the Dazaifu headquarters from 1228 until he died from wounds suffered in the second Mongol invasion of Japan in 1281. With Sukeyoshi's backing, Guoming superintended the construction of Jōtenji 承天寺, the first purpose-built Song-style Zen temple erected in Japan. The extent of the religious and trade links established by Guoming is highlighted by the fact that when Wanshou Chanshi burned down in 1242, at Enni's request Guoming shipped a thousand planks of quality lumber from Japan to China as a donation to help in the reconstruction.[18]

Enni's next notable move was to Tōfukuji 東福寺, a Song-style temple complex being built in Kyoto by the aristocrat Kujō Michiie (1193–1252). Of interest here is that Enni assembled a library designed to serve the intellectual interests of Japanese monks who considered themselves Song Zen Buddhists. Thanks to an inventory drawn up by a disciple immediately after Enni's death in 1280, we learn that twenty-nine of the

339 titles were medical works. They are cataloged in four sections and fall into two groups. One group of eleven appears to be pre-Song titles previously held in Japan. The eighteen in the other group appear to be Song titles newly brought to Japan, presumably under Enni's auspices. Not all titles can be fully identified, and four are mentioned twice, but the inventory allows a glimpse of the Song medical knowledge being introduced into Japan at this time.[19]

The titles in the first group are cataloged together and seem to be handwritten scroll copies. Two or possibly three are Chinese works, including an illustrated guide to acupuncture (*Mingtangtu* 明堂図 Bright Hall Illustrated), and the *Zhenzhong fang* 枕中方 (Formulas Kept by the Pillow) of the Tang physician Sun Simiao 孫思邈. These would have been either original Tang Chinese manuscripts or Japanese copies of the originals. Two works appear to be Japanese compilations. One, *Yōketsushō* 要穴抄 (Treatise on Prime Insertion Points), may have been a copy of a Heian period moxibustion manual, and the other, *Yakushō* 薬抄, was probably a working reference work. It is unlikely that Enni owned any of these works and more likely that they were provided by Tōfukuji's patron, Kujō Michiie, heir to a family library built up over several centuries.[20] Four other works are formularies. It is unclear if they are Chinese or Japanese ones or a combination of both. One deals with external injury 外境, another with diabetes 消渇飲水, while two, *Zatsuzatsu hō/Zaza fang* 雑々方 (Assorted Formulas) and *Kazō hihō/Jiacang mifang* 家蔵秘方 (Secret Formulas from Family Treasuries), are general handbooks.

The titles in the second group are all Song printed books. Some are (probably Northern) Song editions of classic works, such as the *Huangdi neijing*'s *Suwen jing* 素問経 (Canon of Basic Questions); two works on pulse diagnosis, *Wang Shuhe maijue* 王叔和脉訣 (Wang Shuhe's Secrets of Pulse) and *Tong Zhenzi maijue* 通眞子脉訣 (Tong Zhenzi's Secrets of Pulse); and the *Mingtangtu jing* 明堂図経 (Bright Hall Illustrated Canon) on acupuncture. There are also three works on materia medica. One is an illustrated work, another is an explanation of essentials, and the third is an abbreviated guide. Also listed are two late Northern Song works, Zhu Gong's 朱肱 *Shanghan huorenshu* 傷寒活人書 (Book on Keeping People Alive from Cold Damages) of 1108, and Chen Shiwen's 陳師文 *Taiping huimin Hejiju fang* 太平恵民和剤局方 (Formulas of the Pharmacy Service for Great Peace and for the Benefit of the People) of c. 1110. Rounding out the titles are four privately printed formularies from the Southern Song: Xu Shuwei's 許叔微 *Puji benshi fang* 普済本事方 (Effective Formulas for Universal Relief) of c. 1150, Guo Tan's 郭坦 *Shibian liangfang* 十便良方 (Ten Usefulnesses and Effective Formulas) of 1196, Wang Shuo's 王碩 *Yijian fang* 易簡方 (Easy Formulas) of the early 1200s, and Wei Xian's 魏峴 1227 *Weishi jiacang fang* 魏氏家蔵方 (Mr. Wei's Formulas from the Family Storehouse). Whether these titles were selected by Enni (he appears to have had an interest in medicine) or were recommended to him, they seem to have been chosen by someone familiar with the contours of Southern Song medicine. And, since Enni may not have known what medical works were available in Japan or knew that so few were, these titles may have been seen as the core of a monastic medical collection.

To what end might these books have been put at Tōfukuji, apart from taking up space in a library? For Tōfukuji, two areas of activity for which they would have been useful can be identified. First, the Tōfukuji Temple complex was one of the centers for the cult of the Mañjuśrī Bodhisattva, which, as we shall see presently, placed great store on assisting the bereft in society. In addition to addressing spiritual needs, it provided charitable assistance and medical treatment.[21] Since Tōfukuji was located close to one of the more well-known concentrations of the downtrodden (beggars, lepers, outcasts) in Kyoto, it is safe to assume that assistance would have been given to this community. Second, we know that as a matter of course, monks were concerned about their health (mental and physical); in fact, from the earliest days of Buddhism in India, monasteries and temples had always housed specialists who could address the medical needs of the community.[22] Thus, as a matter of course, Tōfukuji's monks would have had more than a casual interest in medicine. Indeed, the 1280 inventory conveys that sense. It notes that *Zatsuzatsu hō/Zaza fang* (Assorted Formulas) and *Kazō hihō/Jiacang mifang* (Secret Formulas from Family Treasuries) are jumbled up and ripped apart, which in context would seem to suggest frequent handling rather than poor storage. Over time, enough Tōfukuji monks trained as physicians that some have identified a "Tōfukuji lineage" of medicine.

This Tōfukuji lineage—or at least people who had become acquainted with its medical activities while staying there—was also a link in a wider Buddhist network through which medical knowledge was disseminated. One of the key insights into how this might work is provided by Kajiwara Shōzen. In his *Man'anpō,* he notes the following:

> With respect to this medicine [the Yu Family Meeting the Transcendent Pill 兪家遇仙丹]: the Buddhist monk Dōshō of Jisshō-in 實相院 Temple in Mikawa Province resided in China for nine years in order to learn and have transmitted to him the medical arts. He received the transmissions for such formulas as Black Tin Pill 黒錫丹, Nourishing Life Pill 養生丹, and Spirit Sand Pill 霊砂丹; for the oral transmissions for pulse analysis, acupuncture, and moxibustion; and for this Meeting the Transcendent Pill. Monk Dōshō then transmitted it to Zen Master [Mujū] Ichien (the elder at Owari Province's Chōboji Temple) since [Ichien] had such a great interest in all things associated with Buddhism. Then Zen Master Ichien transmitted it to his brother Jisshō 實照, and Jisshō further transmitted it to me, Shōzen. In the Song this formula has been a secret of the Yū's lineage and has not been transmitted to any other families. It is strictly guarded and had not been known in Japan. Thusly it was transmitted in the lineage of Zen Master Dōshō, and it has come into my hands. Our descendants must maintain this as secret.[23]

This and other information gives us a picture something like the following. Dōshō is the first Japanese monk known to have gone to China for the express purpose of studying medicine, and he spent nine years there sometime between the mid-1240s and late 1250s. He studied under the Yu lineage of physicians, received extensive training in a range of healing methods, and was taught at least one other special formula in addition to the ones listed by Shōzen.[24] Dōshō appears to have been a disciple of Enni Ben'en. Jisshō-in Temple had been founded by Enni, and only someone with a strong connection to him would have been able to become its head. Too, since Dōshō seems to have gone to China subsequent to Enni's return, there is a strong likelihood that Enni encouraged him to study medicine in China: The topics that Dōshō studied and his knowledge of formulas overlap substantially with the titles in the Tōfukuji inventory.

After his return from China, Dōshō was resident for some time at Tōfukuji, and we may assume that he shared his new knowledge of acupuncture, moxibustion, and formulas with fellow monks. One of the monks with whom he interacted was Mujū Ichien (1226–1312), an eclectic figure who had studied in Kamakura Zen temples before going to Tōfukuji to study under Enni. Ichien's interests in medicine are separately attested in his writings (such as the *Shasekishū* 砂石集, A Collection of Sand and Pebbles), and at some point prior to 1263, Dōshō imparted knowledge of

Meeting the Transcendent Pill to Ichien. Later, when resident at a temple about halfway between Kyoto and Kamakura, Ichien passed that information to his brother (whether a biological or a religious brother is not clear) Jisshō. Jisshō then passed the lore to Shōzen, a monk who practiced medicine in Kamakura and belonged to the Ritsu Precept sect. Ichien and Shōzen (and possibly Jisshō) were also members of the Kajiwara warrior clan of Sagami Province, in which the city of Kamakura was located.[25] It may be that Dōshō told others of the Meeting the Transcendent Pill and that they in turn conveyed it further, since even from this one example it is evident that information flowed through a web of connections.

By the time Shōzen wrote down this Chinese formula in the *Manan'pō* in the 1320s, it had been in circulation among Japanese Buddhist monks for around seventy years. It is entirely likely that this example of the Meeting the Transcendent Pill was not an isolated case but representative of general practices. For example, a source dated to 1326 reveals that a monk who had studied in China brought back with him three special formulas initially produced at several locations; one village that had compounded them gained special distinction. In 1330, the noted prelate Mingji Chujun 明極楚俊 (1262–1336) brought no less than eleven medicines with him to Japan, the compounding technique for one of which, Penetrating Chestnut Powder 通栗散, was subsequently transmitted as a secret tradition. In a slightly different vein, Japanese monks traveling in China, some of whom became seriously ill, were exposed to Chinese physicians and medicines in the normal course of their daily lives. One can easily imagine that some at least would have learned more about these effective medicines and passed on that knowledge to others.[26]

In short, Buddhist monks enjoyed access to Chinese printed books, techniques of treatment, and medicinal formulas. Information about medicines circulated among monks over long distances and extended periods of time. Let us now look at another link in our chain of Buddhist connections, the cult of the Mañjuśrī Bodhisattva and the Ritsu Precept sect, which provided the facilities for Shōzen to engage in his medical activity.

THE BUDDHIST RITSU SECT AND MEDICAL FACILITIES IN KAMAKURA

The Ritsu Precept sect emerged in the thirteenth century against the backdrop of an increase in the numbers and greater visibility of the socially marginalized.[27] Many of these people, the subject of considerable scholarly attention, were referred to by such terms as "Riverbank Dwellers" *(kawaramono)* or "Non-persons" *(hinin).* Contemporary pictorial works, such as the *Ippen shōnin eden* 一遍上人絵伝 (Illustrated Scroll of Holy Man Ippen), reveal that many suffered from hunger, were poorly clothed and housed, received little attention when sick, and included among their numbers those who were physically disabled and those suffering from such medically and socially debilitating ailments as leprosy. They eked out a miserable existence and had to make their way through life with minimal family or social support. Some religious figures, inspired by their understanding of the fundamental Buddhist injunction to end suffering and to heal, sought ways to address their poor living conditions and illnesses. The efforts to do so fell into two basic categories. The first was the provision of some form of relief for people where they were found. The second combined elements of the first with permanent relief and treatment sites.

The first category is exemplified by the activities of the salvation teacher Ippen (1239–1289). As depicted in the *Ippen shōnin eden,* Ippen and his followers regularly distributed food and perhaps provided clothing as well. It is not clear what type of medical assistance, if any, Ippen or those associated with him were able to render, although the charismatic Ippen was seen to possess such a special essence that his urine was believed to be a panacea medicine for myriad ailments. On the other hand, it has been argued that salvational activity itself may constitute a type of medicine, so one might usefully recognize that the assistance rendered and the expression of care had at least a positive impact on people's state of mind (an important consideration in Buddhist healing).[28] Yet, while no doubt those who received Ippen's charity would have been grateful for it, the activity does not appear to have been sustained or regularized.[29]

The second category is exemplified by the activities of the Ritsu Precept sect, which drew its inspiration from the figure of the Mañjuśrī Bodhisattva, who had vowed to help the bereft in society.[30] Just who the bereft are is memorably spelled out in a document from 1267. While the phrasing draws inspiration from Mañjuśrī-related texts and the afflictions are often mentioned in didactic Buddhist writings, it seems to have resonated with conditions in contemporary society:

> Then there are the deaf, blind, and mute, or those with leprosy and boils. They have impediments to hearing the dharma and no means of speech; or their limbs are rotting and falling off, and they have no one

> to treat their ills. The eyes of others are dark and shut tight, and they have no companion to show them the way. When they beg for food and drink from the high and the low, they are despised and arouse feelings of disgust. When they search for scraps of cloth in the wilds, their bodies tire and they cannot go on. The walls of their small shacks are torn, and the mountain storms pierce their skin. The roofs of their grass huts are in disarray, and the evening frost splits their flesh. Never reflecting on the workings of past karma, they resent in vain the harsh workings of humanity. Never considering their extreme suffering in the future, they long only for food and clothing in the present. Don't they realize that due to the grave sin of slandering the Mahayana, they incur the torment of the ten directions' Avīci Hell? And that, because of the gravest, incessant residual karma, they catch the serious disease of human's leprosy? If they do not repent in this life, the future will surely be the same. What could be more lamentable than this?[31]

Assuaging the hunger of the solitary and lepers accorded with Mañjuśrī's salvific powers. The Ritsu Precept sect, under the guidance of its founder Eison (1201–1290), his leading disciple Ninshō (1217–1303), and successors, provided food, clothing, and medical treatment to the disadvantaged on a continuous basis for many decades.[32] Sometimes this occurred in concert with the dedication of a Mañjuśrī votive image, especially at a temple or a location close to the *hinin* outcast communities. As many as three thousand *hinin* might be in attendance on such occasions (the first recorded was in 1240), and each was provided with useful daily items such as straw hats, straw mats, fans, shallow pans, needle and thread, nestled bowls, rice cakes, a lunch box, cloth to use as head covering, broth, mandarin oranges, and water.[33]

Concerns about the bereft in society, particularly in the city of Kamakura, were shared by the leadership of the Kamakura warrior government. By the 1250s, Kamakura had become a crowded urban center beset by a wide range of problems: arson, assault, and random armed violence; overcrowding; unlicensed commercial activity; and a perceived decline in ethical standards among both lay and religious. There also appears to have been a chronic problem with a vagrant *hinin* population. A source from 1221 alludes to a thousand *hinin,* and the number had grown so much by mid-century that twice, in 1247 and 1250, the *bakufu* tried unsuccessfully to drive them out of the city.[34] The concern with *hinin* continued, though a set of ordinances issued in 1261, the New Administrative Regulations, suggest that the attitude towards them and the unfortunate in general had changed. In addition to directing that, for example, prisoners in jail were to be fed and that the buying and selling of human beings was to cease,[35] the regulations note the following:

> Item: The abandoning of the sick, of the solitary and orphaned, and of dead bodies by the roadside, shall be prohibited. When the abandonment of the sick, the solitary and orphaned and such by the roadside is observed it is to be stopped. In cases where they have already been abandoned, then the matter shall be attended to by ward commissioners. The [abandoned] are to be sent to the Mujōdō. Corpses, and the bones and bodies of oxen and horses, are to be taken away.[36]

While it was not unknown for public authority in Kyoto to issue proclamations addressing similar issues,[37] the regulations suggest that the *bakufu*'s concern was not a symbolic one. In fact, the instruction that the abandoned be sent to the Mujōdō suggests that at least one site was already designated as something of a welfare facility.

The concern with the disadvantaged reflected such factors as the individual religious journeys of *bakufu* leaders, their desire to see Kamakura develop as a center of Buddhist culture, and a desire to promote worthy Buddhist behavior.[38] The construction in the 1240s and 1250s of the Kamakura Great Buddha, the second-largest metal cast statue ever constructed in Japan (the largest being the massive Buddha at Tōdaiji in Nara), had been one product of those factors.[39] Another one had been the cooperation between the shogunal regent Hōjō Tokiyori 北条時頼 (1227–1263) and the Chinese monk Lanxi Daolong 蘭渓道隆 (1203–1278), which—with the completion of Kenchōji 建長寺 Zen Temple in 1252—ensured the successful implantation of Song-style monastic Zen Buddhism in Japan.[40] And from the late 1250s, yet another product was the support extended to the Ritsu Precept sect by Tokiyori's uncle and co-regent Shigetoki 北条重時 (1198–1261) and Shigetoki's nephew Kanezawa Sanetoki 金沢実時 (1224–1276). Shigetoki is well known for his two essays on the ethos of warrior leadership, the second of which, written after he had retired to Gokurakuji Temple, is informed by a profound Buddhist worldview.[41] Sanetoki was an avid collector of Song printings of Chinese classics, histories, and religious texts, and he housed his collection (later the Kanazawa

Library) in the precincts of his family temple Shōmyōji 称名寺. In time, both Gokurakuji and Shōmyōji became Ritsu temples. Shōmyōji was particularly attracted to Song culture: It followed Song-style precept observances, and some Shōmyōji heads had their portraits painted in the style of Song Zen masters.[42]

By 1261, the date of the regulations, Sanetoki had established links with two important Ritsu Precept figures. The first figure, Jōshun, had been active in eastern Japan early in his career and spent four years in China in the 1240s. In 1261 he made two book-purchasing trips to China and acquired (among other things) two complete sets of the printed seven-thousand-volume Chinese Buddhist corpus, the *Issaikyō* 一切経. He gave one to Eison and the other to Sanetoki.[43] The second figure, Ninshō, had been active around Kamakura from 1257. Initially based at a temple near Shōmyōji, in 1261 he was made resident priest of a newly converted Ritsu Precept temple in Kamakura, possibly at Sanetoki's behest. Later that year he was charged with saying bedside prayers for the ailing Tokiyori, and in the eleventh month he presided over Shigetoki's funeral. Then in the twelfth month, Sanetoki had Jōshun convey an invitation to Eison to visit Kamakura, which he accepted. Staying along the way at Mujū Ichien's temple of Chōboji, Eison arrived in Kamakura in early 1262. He remained there for six months, engaging in various ritual activities and social works and interacting with prominent Kamakura figures.[44] Ninshō was also in Kamakura at this time and engaged in good works. He provided food to beggars; distributed offerings received at religious ceremonies to beggars, sufferers from skin diseases, and prisoners; and he distributed food to people at a lodging facility for victims of leprosy.[45] Soon after Eison's departure, Tokiyori invited Ninshō to lecture on Buddhism, and Shigetoki's second son, Hōjō Naritoki (1242–1287), invited him to become resident at another temple.

By 1267, Ninshō had assumed the headship of the late Shigetoki's Gokurakuji Temple, which had now become a Ritsu Precept sect temple.[46] At Gokurakuji, Ninshō became the face of public welfare in Kamakura, and the Gokurakuji administrative office oversaw the logistics of that activity.[47] The Hōjō allocated permanent resources such as property rights transferred from their own extensive portfolio of holdings to support those activities. In addition, the Hōjō gifted Gokurakuji trade management privileges in Kamakura and in Hakata, and on at least one occasion Gokurakuji was cosponsor of a trade ship to China sent to gain funds for temple reconstruction.[48] Ninshō was well aware of the fruits of the China contact. Though he had been refused permission to travel to China, in 1248 he was dispatched to Hakata to personally escort the bulk of the printed texts that Jōshun had acquired in China to Eison's headquarters at Saidaiji Temple 西大寺.[49]

What were some of the ways the money was used? We do not have information on day-to-day activities, but we do have some references to times of large-scale emergency need. For example, in 1264 Ninshō distributed food to three thousand *hinin* in Kamakura. During a famine in 1274, he assembled the starving at a spacious area near the Kamakura Great Buddha, at Daibutsugatani, and distributed rice soup for over fifty days; we might reasonably assume that this involved providing thousands if not tens of thousands of meals. And during an epidemic in 1283, Ninshō provided food and sustenance at the entrance to Gokurakuji Temple.

Another activity was of arguably greater importance. Under Ninshō's leadership, Gokurakuji established a substantial public medical treatment facility. The facility established in 1287 at Kuwagatani was perhaps the most sophisticated and extensive medical facility in Japanese history to that time (and probably for many centuries thereafter).[50] A later map of Gokurakuji identifies a Hall of the Medicine Buddha 薬師堂, a clinical treatment building, a lodging for leprosy *(rai)* sufferers, a medicinal bathhouse, a dispensary for medicines, a lodging for the ill, an equine veterinary clinic, and at least one other medical building whose precise function is left unspecified.[51] These facilities would have required a wide range of personnel: physicians; people to assist with nursing and perhaps hospice care; people responsible for sanitation, laundry, and cooking; scribes; and purchasing and supply agents for materia medica, food, clothing, writing materials, and assorted implements. Presumably, medical works would also have been kept on hand.

Two contemporary sources shed some light on the scope of the enterprise.[52] The first source informs us that in the thirty-four-year period from 1283 to 1317, a total of 88,167 people were treated at the facilities, of whom 17,168 died and 70,999 were returned to their families. The second source tells us that, in an unspecified twenty-year period, treatment was provided to 57,250 people suffering from *rai;* of these, 10,450 died and 46,800 were successfully treated.[53] If we take these figures at face value, then the first source suggests that on average, 2,593 patients were treated each year, of whom 505 died and 2,088 were returned to their families; of the average

239 patients treated each month, 44 died and 195 were returned to their families. From the second source, noting 57,250 *rai* sufferers treated over a twenty-year period, we get an average annual number of 2,862 people receiving treatment, of whom 522 died and 2,340 were successfully treated. Of the average 246 patients treated in the course of a month, 43 died and 203 were treated successfully.

Obviously, these figures need to be treated with caution. We do not know whether they refer to distinct individuals or whether they refer to instances (which might mean an individual is counted more than once); we do not know whether the higher figure of 88,167 includes *rai* sufferers or whether (as in the second source) figures for *rai* sufferers may have been kept separately; averages give us no guide to actual rhythms of treatment; and we do not know what relationship there may be between successful treatment and returning people to their families. However, since Kamakura's population by the late 1200s is estimated at between 50,000 and 100,000, and Gokurakuji was a treatment center intended to attract the needy, we might reasonably accept the two figures as indicating that at the minimum, somewhere around 250 separate cases were treated on average each month for a period of decades.

In short, Gokurakuji housed a significant medical facility. It enjoyed access to elite patronage. It had the economic wherewithal to support its activities and services. It had regular contact with traders and travelers, who themselves were in continuous contact with sources of knowledge and supplies both within Japan and more broadly throughout East Asia. The physicians who worked at Gokurakuji, such as Kajiwara Shōzen, thus had access to substantial resources, would have enjoyed the opportunity for sustained professional clinical activity, and benefited from a climate that encouraged contact with China.

SHŌZEN'S COSMOPOLITAN KAMAKURA

In 1180, Kamakura was still a small fishing village. By 1185 it had become not only the first new city to be laid out in four hundred years but also the capital of an autonomous warrior administration whose emergence had shattered the monopoly on political power previously enjoyed by the aristocracy. Yet while throughout the Kamakura period we see a steady expansion of Kamakura's national authority, the basic policy of the Kamakura regime was that it would benefit more by working in concert with Kyoto rather than against it. Despite structural frictions, it sought to maintain existing administrative and legal structures rather than undermine them.

Nonetheless, by the 1220s the second postfounding generation of warrior leadership had emerged. That leadership was exercised by Japan's first warrior dynasty, the Hōjō family, whose ascent was an unprecedented display of upward mobility. The Hōjō were to control Kamakura until its demise in the 1330s. Having being raised in an environment of warrior supremacy—and also eager to establish their own social and cultural credentials—the second-generation Hōjō were determined to shape Kamakura as a religious and cultural center distinct from the imperial capital. It is probably fair to say that they saw Kamakura as Japan's alternative capital. The Hōjō were aware that to build a Kamakura culture, they would not be able to look to Kyoto for either support or inspiration: The aristocracy was loath to share any of its cultural capital with its social inferiors, and the Hōjō did not want their city to be merely an imitation of Kyoto's culture. Accordingly, they were receptive to new possibilities.

The Kamakura mind-set was outward looking. Whereas the wealth of the old aristocracy derived from control over land rights—and indeed, land rights remained the basic form of wealth in warrior society—Kamakura had a positive attitude towards the accumulation of wealth through trade and commerce. The Hōjō desire to build up wealth and resources where none had existed before reflected the need to firmly establish itself as preeminent. They also needed to ensure that tax-rice and bulk goods from throughout the country, particularly from landholdings located in central and western Japan, would flow directly to Kamakura and not be funneled through the older routes that converged on Kyoto. One tangible result of that concern was the building of the artificial port of Wakaejima in Kamakura's bay in 1232, which also symbolized Kamakura's embrace of maritime commerce. Even in the Sea of Japan, on the opposite side of the main island of Honshu, ships sailed under pennants emblazoned with the Hōjō family crest. The Hōjō also opened up new routes along the Pacific coast that linked Kamakura directly to Hakata and to the China trade. In fact, by the 1220s the old Dazaifu headquarters had become an arm of Kamakura, and the Hōjō had become aware of the rhythms of trade and human activity across and around the East China Sea.

Due to the new shipping routes and to its rapid emergence as Japan's second-largest population center, Kamakura came to resemble Hakata as much as it did the imperial capital—and then some. Hakata, still a vibrant entrepôt, took on a new role as Kamakura's transshipment center for goods flowing to and from China, and Kamakura became the new eastern terminus of the East Asian maritime trade network. In some areas of trade—such as Chinese ceramics—Kamakura even replaced Hakata as a national distribution center.[54] To give a sense of how extensive the ceramic trade was, we only need note some of what was recovered from one Chinese trade ship bound for Hakata that was sunk off the southwestern coast of Korea in 1323. In addition to copper coins, metalwork, red sandalwood, and other items, the cargo included 20,661 pieces of pottery. Most of these were Chinese ceramics produced in kilns in southern Zhejiang Province (12,359 pieces of celadon) and northern Jiangxi Province (5,303 pieces of white ware). The two most common ceramics were the 10,000 double-handled vases and the 3,500 blue and white peony arabesque bottles.[55]

Ceramics were but one type of trade item in a Kamakura fascination with China goods *(karamono)* 唐物, which were carried on China ships *(karabune)* 唐舟. Besides ceramics, the goods included tea, tea utensils, paintings, coins, medicines, fragrances, printed books, large quantities of religious artifacts and religious writings, and (as a by-product) such things as the large six-legged red-lacquered wooden chests that contained the more precious and fragile items. Before the 1180s, eastern Japan had been something of a cultural backwater, but the availability of China goods created a new demand for continental items that only grew throughout the thirteenth century. All segments of the population, not just the elite, eagerly anticipated the arrival of the China ships, and on occasion that eagerness led to disturbances in the city of Kamakura as people vied for them. Evidently these were available in relatively large quantities and sufficiently affordable that many were daily use items rather than prized collectibles. Some items, however, were quite valuable, leading even the *bakufu* leader Kanezawa Sadaaki 金沢貞顕 (1278–1333) to note that they needed to guard against thieves.[56]

The trade was lucrative. On occasion, ships were sent to China in the expectation that the profits—either from Japanese goods shipped to China or from Chinese goods to be sold in Japan, or both—would facilitate repairs of temples or even of Kamakura's Great Buddha.[57] Kamakura's elite families, such as the Kanezawa or the Nikaidō family of officials, actively participated in the China trade.[58] We have few details on individual consignments, but a set of inventories drawn up by the Chinese Zen priest Presider Yi 義首座 following the looting of a becalmed ship by Kyushu coastal residents in 1298 is informative. The ship was Chinese, and the inventory was for luxury goods being sent for trade in China by three apparently well-placed members of Kamakura society. Among the items listed we find gold dust, round gold brick, mercury, swords made of silver or decorated in silver, sets of highly decorated armor with "ark shell" or purple leather binding, a "Chinese-style" monk's surplice, gold- and pearl-decorated swords, gilt-inlaid cutting knives, gold-dust sprinkled tin cosmetic chests, decorated and gold-flecked ablution basins, various types of woven cloth, teacup stands, gold-flecked inkstones, and sacks of pearls.[59]

Presider Yi's role as a *bakufu* envoy charged with recovering valuable goods from Japanese commoners directs us to another element of Kamakura's cosmopolitanism. Namely, it was home to many Chinese (it was also home to many Japanese monks who had lived in China, but I will not pursue this here). We are most familiar with eminent Zen monks (such as Lanxi Daolong) who were active in the latter part of the 1200s, but it is clear that Kamakura's Chinese, while overwhelmingly male and in religious orders, were not limited to a few individuals who are known for their historical impact. Some, like Qingzhuo ōshō 清拙和尚 (1274–1339), who was invited to Kamakura in 1326 by the most powerful warrior of the day, Hōjō Takatoki 北条高時 (1303–1333), and presided over one event that was attended by over a thousand participants, did of course have very public profiles.[60] Others were known for skills in specialty areas, such as Hanzhang and the priest Langyuan *fang*, both of whom were physicians who attended on the *bakufu* leader Hōjō Tokimune 北条時宗 (1251–1284).[61] Another individual, noted only as a Song person 宋人, was the source of a secret transmission for a medicine for a swollen scrotum.[62] The monk Daishi *seng* 大食僧, who was in charge of garden landscaping at Shōmyōji, seems originally to have been a member of an Islamic merchant family resident in south China who had converted to Buddhism.[63] Others made their mark as scribes entrusted with copying religious texts or providing the calligraphy for cast-metal bells, such as Daomiao and Changxin; another copyist, Cihong, also contributed (along with the head of Shōmyōji and the *bakufu* official Nagai Sadahide) a poem in a sequence of Chinese poetry on the intriguing topic of living expenses for exiled Chinese.[64] And among these highly literate Chinese residents, we also find at least two—Daoguang 道廣 and another anonymous Song person—who assisted Shōzen and wrote out the final, clean copies of some of the chapters of his magnum opus, the *Man'anpō*.[65]

Finally, let us note some of Shōzen's connections outside of Gokurakuji. We have few sources, but they are instructive. From a notation in the *Man'anpō* from the year 1326, we learn that Shōzen's own handwritten copy of his (no longer extant) three-volume *Hokiron* 補気論 (On Augmenting Qi) was in the possession of Nagai Munehide (fl. 1284–1327) and that another copy was in the library of Nikaidō Yukifuji (1246–1302).[66] Both were powerful members of the *bakufu*'s hereditary bureaucratic elite.[67] Letters written by Munehide's son Sadahide to Myōnin 明忍, then head of Shōmyōji, also make it clear that at least one copy of the *Ton'ishō* was in active circulation.[68] One letter (written in 1308?) notes that he wishes Myōnin to return the copy of the *Ton'ishō* that he had borrowed since someone had expressed a desire to look at it.[69] In another letter, Sadahide notes that he is forwarding the *Ton'ishō* in fifteen sheafs that he wants to borrow, that the work is a wondrous treasure, and that he is also sending along the medicines that Myōnin had requested.[70]

An unsigned letter (from 1325?) is even more revealing.[71] The author of the letter notes that the ointment for boil-sores that the priest-physician Jōkan (i.e., Shōzen) had brought with him and had applied to one Lord Tanaka had worked marvelously. It also reveals that Shōzen was the retainer of Lord Kamon (i.e., Nagai Munehide). Not only does this explain why Munehide might own a copy of the *Ton'ishō,* it also places Shōzen at the center of a network of political patronage that would have given him ready access to Kamakura's bibliographic world centered on Shōmyōji and the Kanazawa Library.

In sum, Shōzen's Kamakura was a vibrant, cosmopolitan city in an era when Japan had launched a new wave of human, cultural, and commercial interaction with China. Kamakura was home to a highly educated Chinese community that was fully integrated into the cultural, political, and intellectual life of the city. Kamakura's ruling elite of warriors and officials was an enthusiastic imbiber of Song Chinese culture and eagerly collected Song printed texts. The warrior leadership also strongly supported the social welfare activities of the Ritsu Precept sect, whose main temple of Gokurakuji also housed the most extensive medical facilities in Japan at that time.

Kajiwara Shōzen was thus eminently well placed. He took advantage of his opportunities to produce two landmark works of medical writing that reflected his own clinical experience and his acquaintance with a wide range of Song medical works. Let us now explore some of the details of that engagement.

Chapter 2

SONG MEDICINE
A View from Japan

This chapter aims to convey a sense of the impact of Song medical texts in medieval Japan by looking at two general themes. The first is how access to Song medical texts restructured the landscape of knowledge about medicine in Japan. For this I examine the background of Japanese medical writing, the scale of Song medical writing, and some of what was learned about medicine from Song writings. The second theme is how some specific elements of knowledge made it possible to identify shortcomings in Japanese medicine and thus to make improvements in Japanese medicine. In taking up these themes, readers will also be able to obtain a broader sense of how Song medicine was understood in early-fourteenth-century Japan.

THE TEXTUAL LANDSCAPE

The Availability of Medical Works

The dearth of Japanese medical works. Prior to the thirteenth century, few works on medicine or on healing were written in Japan, and fewer of them seem to have been in anything like general circulation. Indeed, Kajiwara Shōzen, who was well placed to learn about medical works, mentions few. As far as I can tell, he was completely unacquainted with any work on healing that was associated with the esoteric Tendai and Shingon Buddhist traditions in Japan or any others that advocated ritual healing.

I have been unable to find any Japanese titles in the *Ton'ishō* and only three in the *Man'anpō.* These are Tanba Yasuyori's 丹波康頼 (912–995) *Ishinpō* 医心方 (Formulas from the Heart of Medicine) of 984; Fukane Sukebito's 深根輔仁 *Honzō wamyō* 本草和名 (Japanese Handbook of Materia Medica, early 900s); and Renki's 蓮基 *Chōsei ryōyōhō* 長生療養方 (Formulas for Fostering Long Life) of 1184. The *Chōsei ryōyōhō* is mentioned once and the *Ishinpō* only twice.[1] Either he thought very little of them, or he did not have access to complete copies of them. The *Honzō wamyō,* on the other hand, seems to have been more readily available as a fundamental reference tool, and he refers to it frequently when identifying materia medica. To sum this up, Shōzen seems to have had full access to only one Japanese medical work. What might account for this?

As noted in the previous chapter, the Heian aristocracy set great store in its cultural capital. It is evident that its predilection was for confirming knowledge rather than testing it and for holding knowledge close rather than sharing it. What we know of the Tendai and Shingon sects suggests that they too were secretive. It is perhaps not surprising then that the two main hereditary families of court physicians, the Wake 和気 and the Tanba, had a similar outlook. They were reluctant to divulge titles of medical works in their possession to outsiders. Control of materials was integral to privilege within the families, access to originals and the right to make copies was highly restricted, and careful records were kept on who had read, borrowed, or copied a text.[2] Naturally enough, these restrictions applied to the *Ishinpō.*

We know the *Ishinpō* as one of only two works compiled in Japan prior to the fourteenth century providing comprehensive coverage of medicine. As the original text of the other one, *Daidō ruijūhō* 大同類聚方 (Classified Formulas of the Daidō Era), is no longer extant, *Ishinpō* is thus a medical landmark of great cultural importance. Written on scrolls, it draws on a large number of Sui and Tang period Chinese medical texts, of which the author Yasuyori most likely had direct knowledge. Since only about 5 percent of them are extant, virtually none have survived in China, and many are known only because they are mentioned in the *Ishinpō,* the *Ishinpō* is particularly valued by scholars today for what it tells us of the early Chinese medical tradition.[3] However, this later importance of the *Ishinpō* to Chinese medical bibliography was not known contemporaneously. So what was the *Ishinpō* in the Heian period?

The *Ishinpō* is divided into thirty chapters. It covers such topics as the essence of medicine, acupuncture, eye problems, throat afflictions, pediatrics, obstetrics, sexual techniques, and much more. The *Ishinpō* became the Tanba's core medical text and an embodiment of their cultural capital. It was the major source for subsequent works produced by members of the Tanba family, such as Tanba Masatada's 丹波雅忠 *Iryakushō* 医略抄 (Summary Handbook on Medicine, 1081), or Tanba Yukinaga's 丹波行長 *Eisei hiyōshō* 衛生秘要抄 (Secret Essentials for Safeguarding Life, 1288), a guide to health, longevity, and sexual practices for males produced for a leading political figure. Yet it is not entirely clear that the *Ishinpō* as a consolidated work had an impact on medicine outside of the Tanba family (apart, of course, from whatever effect the treatments drawn from it had on patients). The *Ishinpō* is mentioned in a national bibliographic register in 1293, but few copies appear to have been known to outsiders prior to the fourteenth century. Adding to the rarity of *Ishinpō,* it appears that additional copies of it were made only occasionally, despite the obvious risks to the preservation of knowledge thereby entailed. Finally, and perhaps understandably, since Yasuyori's achievement was so highly regarded, there were no known efforts to revise, expand, or provide a successor text to the *Ishinpō.* In sum, for a number of reasons, the knowledge contained in the *Ishinpō* was restricted, highly regarded, and preserved—but perhaps also ossified.[4]

So, if we take the *Ishinpō* as an example, then the other works produced by the Tanba would not have circulated widely either. It seems that the same is true for works produced by other court physicians. For example, in the 1280s Koremune Tomotoshi 惟宗具俊 compiled his *Honzō iroha shō* 本草色葉鈔 (Materia Medica in Japanese Alphabetical Order, c. 1284). This was a systematic guide to variant Chinese nomenclature for materia medica based on painstaking cross-referencing of the *Daguan bencao* 大観本草 (Daguan Era Materia Medica, c. 1108)[5] and is more voluminous than the *Honzō wamyō.* Yet it is not listed in the register of books held in Japan that was compiled in 1293. And Shōzen was totally unaware of it.

In short, while further study of the topic might lead me to qualify these remarks subsequently, it is very hard to avoid the conclusion that the textual horizons of Japanese medicine were limited. Not many works were produced, access to them was highly restricted, and those in possession of them do not seem to have been at all motivated to share their knowledge. The Song environment was quite different.

The Song information revolution. The development of wood-block printing in the Song dynasty ushered in a revolution in the production, dissemination, reproduction, and preservation of information. Whereas prior to this time, reproduction of a work required time-consuming and laborious transcription by hand to create one scroll copy at a time, the advent of wood-block printing meant that the only practical limit on reproducing a work was the condition of the woodblocks and the demand for the item. Copies could now be produced quickly and never ran the risk of transcription error, and reprints could be made over an extended period of time. Moreover, the change in format—from scroll to book—made works more portable: Quite apart from issues of size, many formerly separate physical scrolls could now be combined as sections of a larger physical work (of course, titles might still be produced in what we understand as multivolume works). In addition, the ease of printing encouraged large-scale projects, such as a standard edition of the 5,048-volume edition of the Buddhist *Tripitika* 大蔵経 (first printed in 972–983) or the consolidation of knowledge in the thousand-volume *Taiping yulan* (Imperial Digest of the Taiping Era, completed in 977, first printed early in the next century). Finally, printing transformed the production of knowledge into a more complex enterprise. An industry was created where none had existed before, and it combined such elements as composition, carving of woodblocks, printing, editing, proofreading, bookbinding, and distribution into an integrated process. Large projects required large resources, and often only government support made them possible. But with the gradual development of a commercial book industry, the issue of cost for an individual author may have become less of an issue.

While it is likely that only a portion of the total number of works written during the Song ended up being printed, the print revolution created a new world for the production and consumption of knowledge. Material became available in ways that had not been possible before. Self-publishing created its own dynamic. Printed material could be disseminated to a wider audience, even to distant locations of which the author might be totally unaware. The print revolution also enabled individuals and institutions, no longer constrained by cost or the rarity of handwritten scrolls, to consider becoming collectors of books and creating libraries that contained a broad range of materials. Also, the prestige attendant upon owning a collection of printed works no doubt gave books a value beyond their specific content.

In sum, wood-block printing created an information revolution. As is well known, it had a significant impact in such areas as education, the examination system, and on the technology of civil administration. The impact on medical knowledge was no less transformative.

Rhythms of medical printing in Northern and Southern Song. As far as I am aware, the best available estimate is that approximately 150 medical works are known to have been printed in the roughly 350-year period during which the Northern Song, Southern Song, Jin, and Yuan dynasties ruled all or parts of China.[6] However, since the works available in Japan were primarily ones produced in the Northern and Southern Song and since medical writing in the Yuan may be seen as a continuation of trends already evident, I will focus my comments on the Song eras. Also, since the 150 works include those preserved outside China but not in China, it is reasonable to assume that there were other works printed that left no trace, so the total number may have been higher than 150. In any event, the extant works are sufficient to permit us to suggest the rhythms of production and the characteristics of medical works printed during this long period.

The Northern Song gave great attention to rebuilding the written heritage and then adding to it.[7] With respect to medicine, this involved three broad areas of activity: making corrections to older reference works, creating standard editions of classic works, and compiling new works under imperial auspices. Much of this work was carried out by officials working in official editing organizations, such as the Bureau for Emending Medical Texts 校正医書局. The first area, the concerted effort to standardize knowledge of materia medica, involved two main elements: rectifying inaccuracies that had crept into the written pharmacopoeia and, as far as possible, gathering existing knowledge of materia medica and formulas so that they might be incorporated as appropriate into the new edited editions. One example of this is the twenty-volume *Kaibao xinxiang ding bencao* 開宝重定本草 (Kaibao Era Newly Edited and Revised Pharmacopoeia). The second area, creating standard editions of classic works, involved deciding what they were, discovering extant copies, and identifying variant versions. The search was wide ranging. For example, it was discovered that works no longer known in China were preserved in Korean collections, and they were then reintroduced into the Chinese medical corpus. Perhaps the clearest measure of the importance of this recovery project is that no editions of the classic works that predate those produced under the Song are known to us; that is, the Song editions are the oldest versions of record. Among the works recovered were the *Huangdi neijing suwen* (Huangdi Internal Classic Basic Questions) on acupuncture, the third-century *Shanghan lun* 傷寒論 (Treatise on Cold Damage) of Zhang Zhongjing 張仲景, and the Tang-era *Beiji qianjin yaofang* 備急千金要方 (Priceless and Essential Formulas for Emergencies) of Sun Simiao 孫思邈. However, the recovery of the works could involve so much editorial attention that an entirely new work was created. A good example of this is Zhang Zhongjing's *Jingui yaolüe fanglun* 金匱要略方論 (Synopsis of Formulas from the Golden Chamber).[8] The third area of activity, producing new works, resulted in the appearance of such titles as the hundred-volume *Taiping Shenghui fang* 太平聖惠方 (Formulas of Great Peace and Sagely Benevolence; hereafter, *Shenghui fang*) of 992 with its 16,834 formulas; the *Jiayou buzhu bencao* 嘉祐補注本草 (Jiayou Era Annotated Materia Medica) of 1062; and the early-twelfth-century *Taiping huimin Hejiju fang* (Formulas of the Pharmacy Service for Great Peace and for the Benefit of People; hereafter *Hejiju fang*).

In the Southern Song, in contrast to the government-sponsored activity of the Northern Song, printed medical literature tended to be produced by private individuals. I shall comment on a number of these works presently, so it is worth noting the salient characteristics of Southern Song medical printing suggested by Kosoto Hiroshi.[9] First, the printing was decentralized. Second, there was nothing like a unified editorial thrust, by which I mean that we cannot identify for the Southern Song any particular projects or overall vision behind the appearance of any works. Third, the works were produced by a variety of physicians and interested amateurs (such as a failed examination candidate, a well-placed official, or someone who had survived a smallpox epidemic). The printing costs were met variously, including the appropriation of government funds, paying for someone else's work to be published, and funding one's own work. Fourth, reflecting the preceding, while some works were highly regarded by later generations as well as by contemporaries, very few were intended to be part of any official canon. Instead, many were intended as ephemeral working reference manuals. One upshot of all this is that Southern Song works provide a closer sense of the world of contemporary medicine than do the works produced during the Northern Song. It is also clear that there were no inherent restrictions on the circulation of printed works or on the dissemination of the information they contained.

Having sketched what we might regard as the appropriating context of Song medicine, let us now look at some of the works that came to Shōzen's attention.

Chinese Works Noted in the *Ton'ishō* and *Man'anpō*

Some 55 Chinese medical works are noted in the *Toni'shō,* and 273 medical works (plus 3 Japanese medical works, 55 nonmedical works, and 279 individuals) are noted in the *Man'anpō.* Courtesy of an unpublished index to the *Man'anpō,* we further know that titles are mentioned approximately 1,860 times, authors and individuals are mentioned on 1,910 occasions, and that the formulas in it were selected from 88 of these titles.[10] While works noted in the *Ton'ishō* also reappear in the *Man'anpō,* it is clear that Shōzen continued to acquire titles subsequent to the completion of the *Ton'ishō.* However, Shōzen did not have direct access to all of the titles that he mentions. As was common in Chinese medical writing, later works often cited earlier works, and so a number of Shōzen's citations are indirect rather than direct references.[11] Nonetheless, it is fairly easy to identify the works to which he had physical access by noting the citations, his comments throughout the text, or when he compares formulas. Since Southern Song works rarely cite each other (this is particularly true of the formula handbooks), it is almost certain that mention of such works means that he had used the original. That said, most of the citations in the *Ton'ishō* and the *Man'anpō* are drawn from only six works, though a much larger number than that were used to augment or provide a comparison with the information in those six.

Using the raw number of formulas listed in the *Ton'ishō* and the *Man'anpō* as a gauge of the relative importance of works, then we discover the following.[12] Of the 1,400 formulas in the *Ton'ishō,* 865 are taken from four works, namely the *Shenghui fang* 聖恵方 (258; the edition used by Shōzen was a printed one of 1147),[13] the *Hejiju fang* (220), the Tang-era *Qianjin fang* 千金方 (Priceless Formulas, 196), and the *Sanyin fang* (first printed in 1174; 191). The next six works upon which Shōzen drew provide a total of 334 formulas. With respect to the 3,100 formulas in the *Man'anpō,* these same four *(Shenghui fang, Hejiju fang, Qianjin fang,* and *Sanyin fang)* contribute fewer formulas (480 total; respectively 217, 156, 84, and 23), but they retain their relative ranking to each other. However, they are dwarfed by the formulas drawn from two works that became available to Shōzen after he completed the *Ton'ishō.*

The first of these, the *Shengji zonglu* 聖済総録 (Comprehensive Record of Sagely Benevolence, compiled 1111–1117), came to Shōzen hot off the presses. Though completed nearly two hundred years earlier, it had effectively become lost and had only become widely known via a Yuan printed edition of 1300 (which was the edition used by Shōzen).[14] Shōzen selected approximately 1,797 formulas from among the 20,000 it contained, thus making it the single most important source of the formulas in the *Man'anpō,* accounting for 60 percent of all of them. These are found in chapters 1 through 38. The second work and the source of the second-largest number of formulas is the pediatrics work *Youyou xinshu* 幼幼新書 (New Pediatrics, first printed in 1150). Picking up where the *Shengji zonglu* left off, *Youyou xinshu* is the dominant source of information and organization for the eleven pediatrics chapters (chapters 39–49), which themselves constitute about 20 percent of the *Man'anpō.* However, the *Youyou xinshu* contains very few of its own formulas and instead draws them from other works. Thus, despite the fact that the *Youyou xinshu* is cited 143 times, few if any formulas are attributed to it.[15] That is, unless attested elsewhere in Shōzen's writings, he probably did not have access to the original works noted in the *Youyou xinshu* and mentioned in these chapters of the *Man'anpō.*

While Shōzen took many formulas from a few works, he also actively selected formulas from other sources that were generally more recent compilations. It is also clear that, while a few works contributed the bulk of the formulas, Shōzen compared those with versions of them in later works and did not simply copy them in without first evaluating them. Two examples involving the *Hejiju fang* and the *Yuyaoyuan fang* 御薬院方 (Formulas of the Imperial Pharmacy Service, c. 1242) may illustrate this. In one case, after listing a formula from the *Hejiju fang,* he notes that the *Yuyaoyuan fang* increases the amount of prepared aconite root.[16] In another case, he observes that the *Yuyaoyuan fang* has built on the formula for Neutralize Food Pill 消食円 by adding a little more of ginseng, poria, and cassia, substituting large barley sprouts for small barley sprouts, and then he has renamed the formula as Thinking of Food Pill 思食円, "which is wonderful."[17]

In using this range of printed medical works, Shōzen provides us with his picture of Song medicine. Since the works to which he had access include both those that survived in China and ones that were not preserved (or much cited) in China after that time, it is possible that he provides a different sense of contemporary Song medicine than is possible from relying just on texts that survived in China. That is, just as the *Ishinpō* preserves a sense of Tang medicine that was lost in China, so too might Shōzen for the Song.

In any event, in addition to the six main works noted above, Shōzen had access to such Song works as the *Puji benshi fang* (Effective Formulas for Universal Relief) of c. 1150, the 1186 *Yeshi luyan fang* 葉氏録験方 (Mr. Ye's Tested Formulas), the 1189 *Yishuo* 医説 (Conversations on Medicine), the 1226 *Huoren shizheng fang houji* 活人事証方後集 (Proven Formulas for Keeping People Alive, Continued), and the 1253 *Yanshi jisheng fang* 巌氏済生方 (Mr. Yan's Formulas for Benefiting Life). He also used Chen Ziming's 陳自明 treatises on gynecology and obstetrics (*Furen daquan liangfang* 婦人大全良方, Complete Effective Formulas for the Diseases of Women, 1237) and on external medicine (*Waike jingyao* Essentials of External Medicine, 1263).[18] In addition he had access to such Yuan works as Xu Guozhen's 許国禎 *Yuyaoyuan fang,* the late-thirteenth-century *Rencun Sunshi zhibing huofa mifang* 仁存孫氏治病活法秘方 (Rencun Mr. Sun's Practical Remedies and Secret Formulas for Treating Illness), and the 1306 *Fengke jiyan mingfang* 風科集験名方 (Famous Effective Formulas for Wind Disorders).

Among the works that disappeared in China and in many cases were preserved only in Japan, we find titles such as the *Yijian fang* 易簡方 (Easy Formulas, early 1200s), the 1178 (second printing 1185) *Yangshi jiacang fang* 楊氏家蔵方 (Mr. Yang's Formulas from the Family Treasury), the 1197 *Shizhai baiyi xuanfang* (Shizhai's 101 Selected Formulas), the 1226 *Beiji jiu fang* 備急灸方 (Emergency Moxibustion Formulas), the 1227 *Weishi jiacang fang* (Mr. Wei's Formulas from the Family Treasury), the 1243 *Xu yijian fang* 続易簡方 (Easy Formulas, Continued), the 1260 (?) *Jianyi fanglun* 簡易方論 (Discourse on Easy Formulas) of the unsuccessful examination candidate Li Minshou 黎民壽. One work, the undated and unattributed *Keyong fang* 可用方 (Indispensable Formulas), which Shōzen mentions an astonishing 251 times in the *Man'anpō* (he comments on the information it contains and formulas drawn from it), is otherwise unattested.

These are formula handbooks that were meant to be contemporary reference works, and they lay no claim to innovation in treatment or theory. That is, while the authors obviously wished to preserve knowledge and to make it more widely available—and may have hoped that some record of their lifework would result—the works are ephemera rather than classics. Nonetheless, Shōzen's use of them indicates that he had a good overall sense of Song medicine as it was in his day. These works were also substantial. For example, Yang Tan's 楊倓 *Yangshi jiacang fang* (Mr. Yang's Formulas from the Family Treasury), which was printed by the author himself at the local county office, ended up in the Kanazawa Bunko Library in Kamakura. It is a work of twenty volumes and fifty-nine topic categories, and contains 1,311 formulas. A second example is Wei Xian's 魏峴 1227 *Weishi jiacang fang* (Mr. Wei's Formulas from the Family Treasury), well regarded in China at least through 1321 (after which it became lost) and housed in Tōfukuji in Kyoto as early as the 1240s.[19] It is organized into twelve volumes and forty-one topical sections, and contains 1,051 formulas that include ones handed down from his grandfather. It also confirms the widespread use of formulas that contain materia medica of non-Chinese (Southeast Asian, Middle Eastern) origin whose inclusion in the pharmacopoeia was, as we will explore in the next chapter, one of the major developments in Song medicine.

A Japanese Snapshot of Song Medicine

Titles of works obviously shed light on topics that are of medical interest. But medical works also convey something of the contours of medicine. What might Shōzen have gleaned? In addressing this, I will not take up issues of nosology and etiology that appear in the introductory sections or in other places throughout his chapters.[20] Instead I will look at what he may have learned about medicine as an area of knowledge and endeavor. After all, he was engaging material of a type that effectively did not exist in Japanese medical writing.

Following are four examples that cover, respectively, a specialized field, medicine provided to the Yuan imperial elite, a work that was obviously grounded in case histories, and the phenomenon of updated or expanded editions.

The first example is a work on women's medicine, the 1237 *Furen daquan liangfang* (Complete Effective Formulas for the Diseases of Women) of Chen Ziming. While not the first specialized treatment of the topic, it is often considered to be the first useful engagement of women's medicine.[21] Ziming, like his predecessors over many centuries, felt that the most difficult area in the medical arts was the treatment of the conditions and symptoms (especially during pregnancy) of women. In his preface he tells us how the work came into being. He notes that his family had been interested in learning about medicine for three generations and had collected a number of works; he had also studied various formulas that he had sought out and examined while traveling, and he selected the best books and augmented these with formulas that had been used in his family and compiled these in one book. He divided the work into eight sections, starting with menstruation and ending with birth; each section records several tens of symptoms, and he has around 260 of his own disquisitions regarding the symptoms. Following each of these, he collated and set down appropriate formulas. It is evident that the work reflected direct personal experience with formulas and with patient responses. Finally, he tells us that all has been organized into an easily understandable form, edited, and then indexed.

The second example is a work that shares the medical knowledge that was used to treat the most powerful people in society, and thus in part it conveys the message that the general population should also benefit from the best medicine. The work is the 1267 *Yuyaoyuan fang* (Formulas of the Imperial Pharmacy Service), authored by Xu Guozhen, offspring of a family of doctors from Shanxi Province. The work is in twenty volumes, divided into fourteen sections (fields of medicine and illness categories), and it contains some 1,059 formulas. It is cited extensively in the *Man'anpō.* It drew its general distinction, particularly after the fall of the Southern Song in 1279, from two factors. First, Xu Guozhen was the long-term personal physician of Khubilai Khan and his wife.[22] Second, it is an authoritative selection of the formulas used by the Yuyaoyuan (Imperial Dispensary), the office responsible under the Song, Jin, and Yuan dynasties for the management and provision of medicines at the imperial court. The work does not suggest any obvious breakthroughs in treatment and may not cover everything that it is possible to cover, but it is a good guide to treatment for the elite and to contemporary medicine in general. The formulas were literally only those that were considered fit for an emperor. They reflect and incorporate the most up-to-date knowledge of materia medica, which knowledge we might reasonably assume to have been drawn from throughout the vast reaches and trading networks of the Mongol Empire(s) as of the 1260s.[23]

The third example is of formula handbooks, which suggest that keeping medical records, sharing the results of one's clinical efforts, and providing evidence of efficacy by citing examples of treatment of actual patients proved more useful to others than the simple listing of formulas. Here I note Xu Shuwei's 許叔微 mid-twelfth-century *Puji benshi fang* (Effective Formulas for Universal Relief).[24] This guide to ailments and treatments was evidently based upon the author's own records and notes, and it provides a close look at aspects of contemporary clinical medicine. The ten volumes and the twenty-six topic sections include discussions of acupuncture and moxibustion and offer the reader three hundred handy formulas. In general, the formulas are ones employed in treating a specific problem and reflect the details of actual case records rather than a more generalized "one size fits all" formula. Thus for itchiness, we encounter separate formulas for such cases as a young boy with pain in both armpits, or for a patient with itchiness and pain in the stomach and armpits. The same approach is evident in sections dealing with aching head and dizziness and for ailments of women and children. The entries provide brief information on the symptoms, details regarding a patient's prior condition, and the formula(s) used in treating the patient. There is the greatest amount of detail for the more complex cases. The style of presentation seems to suggest that the writer is conveying, "This is what I used in this case, and it was successful, thus it is here recorded." That is, there is the sense that what we are reading is the product of clinical testing and experience rather than abstract theoretical engagement of medicine and illness.

The final example, using the *Hejiju fang,* conveys the point that medicine could be amended and expanded. We do not know whether Shōzen (or anyone else for that matter) would be aware of the print history of any work, but he would have discovered something new: namely that it was possible for there to be multiple versions of a work.

Between its first appearance in 1107–1110 and 1252, the *Hejiju fang* went through at least four revisions and expansions.[25] Sometimes it is possible to identify which or how many editions of the *Hejiju fang* an author may have used; we know, for example, that Shōzen's contemporary Koremune Tomotoshi used at least three editions (those of 1108, 1185, and 1195) of the *Hejiju fang* when compiling his *Honzō irohashō.*[26] In Shōzen's case, while it is evident that he was using more than one edition of the *Hejiju fang,* it is not yet clear which ones these were. However, Shōzen knew that he was using different editions and checked them against each other. In one example, when providing information on a *Hejiju fang* formula for Five Fragrance Powder 五香散, Shōzen notes that the "different edition *Jufang*" 別本局方 omits *agastache* and adds musk.[27] Another example suggests that Shōzen may have been using two editions in addition to the one to which he refers by default. He notes that a formula listed in the "different edition" is noted by various newly arrived formularies 新渡諸方 to be a false formula, so he hasn't recorded it; and in the same entry he notes that in the formula for Mr. Guang's Response to Sensations Pill 廣氏感応円, the different edition adds a number of extra ingredients, but as he hasn't written them down in the present entry, the reader wanting to use it should look at the expanded and annotated version of the *Hejiju fang* 增注大全和剤局方.[28] And, in a different vein, having the *Hejiju fang* meant he could identify that a work cited in the *Youyou xinshu* as the *Dayiju fang* 大医局方 (Formulas from the Great Medicine Bureau) was actually the *Hejiju fang* (although he refers elsewhere to at least one formula as a citation from the *Dayiju fang*).[29]

So what are some things he could learn from Song medicine that could not have been readily understood from Japanese medical tradition? For one thing, Shōzen would have gained a sense of the development of particular branches of medicine and also that some works were acknowledged as carrying with them particular medical authority. For example, the *Youyou xinshu* has a listing of those works deemed most significant for that compilation and thus to the field of pediatrics. The listing of eight "former age" 前代 works, forty "recent age" 近世 works, and twenty-five private works provides a sense of old and new in medicine that was unknown in Japan. Shōzen copied this information verbatim.[30]

Another thing that Shōzen would have discovered was that medicine was not a static enterprise, that new views were acceptable, and that they could be employed to advantage. A ready example of this is provided by Chu Yushi's 初虞世 famous, but no longer extant, *Yangsheng biyong fang* 養生必用方 (Essential Formulas for Nurturing Life, 1097). It appears that Shōzen had access to a physical copy and that he was aware of its reputation.[31] This work is not mentioned in the *Ton'ishō,* but it is in the *Man'anpō,* which suggests that it may have come to Shōzen's attention after 1304. The *Man'anpō* includes sixteen formulas from *Yangsheng biyong fang,* Chu's name appears at least forty times, the work is mentioned seventy-seven times, and often when it is cited it is because Shōzen has recourse to its authority in order to make some important points about how approaches to medicine should change.

SHŌZEN'S DISCOVERIES: SONG ADVANCES AND JAPANESE DEFICIENCIES

In addition to what he learned from printed medical texts about medicine as a field of endeavor, Shōzen was also able to learn of new developments in treatment and to evaluate and improve upon aspects of Japanese medical practice. As far as I can tell, Shōzen actively compared older and newer information, cross-checked information in different Chinese works, and selected useful material for clinical application. A number of Shōzen's comments provide us with a window into issues of medicine, illness, and society that, as far as I am aware, have not been noted in other sources (or scholarship).

Comments on Existing Medical Practices and Knowledge

Shōzen provides no readily accessible list or summary that consolidates what he learned of Song and of Japanese medicine as a result of engaging printed medical texts. But throughout the *Ton'ishō* and *Man'anpō,* he makes observations that underscore the breadth of his reading and his clinical experience and that illuminate his discoveries. Quite often these are brief comments. For example, he notes that chest pains affect everybody but that there seems to be a lot of this among women;[32] that there is too much indiscriminate needling and moxibustion;[33] that with respect to vomiting, whereas old medical works sought to treat the problem with warmth medicines, newly arrived works take the position that vomiting arises from heat, and so warming medicines should not be prescribed;[34] and that a newly arrived work provided better information for treating infant and child depression.[35] In another case, he is finally able to identify the condition referred to as imparted illness 継病 (popularly known as *otomi tsuwari*) as infant malnutrition 被鬾 and thus treat it more effectively.[36] Other observations are more substantive and give a better sense of his voice.

Shōzen identified a number of problems with current Japanese medicine that derived from inadequate medical knowledge, bad medical practices, or ignorance. At times, the picture he paints of Japanese medicine—which includes his assessment that Japanese physicians do not consult formula handbooks before they prescribe—is hardly encouraging. Here are some of his comments:

> It is unfortunate that in Japan these days there are those who use cold therapy as well as mistaken needling and indiscriminate moxibustion and cannot discern the rationale for so doing.[37]

> From of old, from the onset of fever related to sore-swellings, in many instances Japanese physicians have used cold water or cold packs and suchlike and given cold therapy. But before the people recovered many of them got apoplexy, suffered cold shakes, and died. This [new Chinese] medicine must be used quickly to ward off the fever. However, treatment must be applied after the patient has dried out [i.e., no longer sweating?].[38]

> I say that with the various swellings, one does not inquire about cold or hot and simply has warming treatments. One must under no circumstances employ cold treatment techniques. These days Japanese physicians do not refer to medical works, but simply in accord with their own opinion they take a wetted stone and forcefully cool [the swelling]. They willfully apply cold treatment, and as a result of this many [patients] get very ill with direct attack of cold or apoplexy, and this leads to painful or sudden deaths. Moreover, the ailing party does not know that the person rendering the treatments is making mistakes. When one thinks about all this, illnesses are the will of Heaven. For heat-toxic swellings there are no theories about [treating them] with cold treatment. How much [more true this is] with cold carbuncles or cold swellings. One must consider this very prudently. In sum, apart from these swellings, we also have toxic swellings, wind swellings, and qi swellings. Their appearance is similar but the treatment is not the same. One must look at volume 135 of the *Shengji zonglu,* as well as volume 7 of the *Keyong fang,* and the second volume of the *Jingyi fang.*[39]

In addition to specific mistakes, Shōzen also identified a major difference in the attitude of Chinese and Japanese physicians towards prescribing medicines. He felt that Japanese physicians were unnecessarily timid in their approach. This may have been related to their lack of familiarity with formula handbooks, to being cautious because their knowledge was limited, or because there was little sense that known formulas might be adjusted. In any event, Shōzen felt that an entirely new attitude was required. In making his case, he felt it useful to harness the authority of the famous Song priest-physician Chu Yushi, author of the *Yangsheng biyong fang.*

> I Shōzen state that for people who are weak and debilitated, one must give a four-type cluster-mix of medicine. Five to six times day and night give medications and meet with them. Even though the person is weak and the medicines strong, one cannot do damage. In recent times,

> patients have been afraid of medicines which are aggressively effective and avoid medications of multiple medicines; simply this strengthens the illness, and conversely if one increases the strength of the medicines this only reduces [its effectiveness?]. This is what Yu Shinan 虞世南 [*sic:* Chu Yushi 初虞世] calls nurturing illness and avoiding treatment. If a person, however, experiences one illness, then numerous illnesses will break out in contention and then one must hurl all kinds of medicines throughout the body. If one gets this import, then one should not be afraid of medicines which are aggressively effective and one should not regard them as the source of weakness in qi. With dispatch, pursue ailments as a soldier pursues an enemy; if one's military might is not continuously applied, then one cannot achieve conquest over the enemy. From the outset, employ Yu Shi[nan]'s import.[40]

> I Shōzen say that doctors in recent times either have fears about administering and mixing many medicines or are afraid of giving many administrations day and night. This is just like fearing medicines and nurturing illnesses. Now the formulas of Yu Shinan [*sic:* Chu Yushi] treat weak people and employ four cluster medicines and advocate six administrations day and night. I think, how can this not be a marvelous injunction![41]

In another example (relating to a formula for infant diarrhea), Shōzen likewise weaves new knowledge, identification of current incorrect information, and important medical authority:

> I say that with respect to poppy capsules, in a certain book it is stated that they greatly harm the spleen and stomach, so it should not be administered to infants and the elderly. For those with robust qi, if one administers medicines containing them then it is very effective. But if one administers it to those with weak qi and who are not eating, then, because they are not eating, it will not be effective. It is also extremely poisonous and not to be casually administered. People of today do not know this and in all types of diarrheas they boil the husks of white mustard seed. As a result, even with young people [their condition] worsens, and even though the diarrhea diminishes, the spleen and stomach are weakened and [the patient] gets the not-eating illness. We see [in the book] that it is not to be given to the elderly or to infants for any length of time. However, when the patient has calmed down and if the spleen

and stomach are settled, then one may compound the medicine and administer a little. But this cannot be given to every person. It is strictly prohibited in the *Daquanliang* [Great Complete Good, *sic*: *Furen daquan liangfang,* The Complete Effective Formulas for Diseases of Women].[42]

Observations on Women's Medicine

Shōzen speaks critically of the state of obstetrics in Japan and provides an intriguing window into matters related to reproduction and childbirth that is not repeated in nonmedical sources and has not been noted by scholars to date. At first glance, we might not associate Buddhist priest-physicians with expertise in matters of reproduction, there perhaps being a presumption that issues of women's health might not be of general interest in a male monastic community. However, Shōzen was a clinical physician at Gokurakuji Temple whose medical mission was to serve all members in society. We know that priest-physicians attended to the medical needs of women who were members of highly placed warrior families, and so we might assume that women of lesser social status would also be among their patients. It is also worth remembering that Shōzen, like many priests, was not celibate and fathered offspring, and so he would have a direct familial interest in medical matters relating to women and children.

The importance of these areas as a medical matter (and, one might infer, as a social matter) is highlighted by the fact that nineteen chapters of the *Man'anpō,* close to one-third of the work, are devoted to obstetrics and pediatrics. This reflects on the one hand the general recognition that the female reproductive experience, from conception through childbirth, was attended by uncertainty and untoward consequences for both mother and child. On the other hand, infant mortality (while we have no figures) appears to have been high, and survival of infants through their first few years was uncertain. It was felt that problems could arise that might not be successfully treatable and where a successful outcome for either or both mother and child was not guaranteed. Thus we find much information regarding such perennial issues as successful nurturing of the fetus, health of the mother, miscarriages, death in childbirth, or infant mortality, as well as ways to nurse the infant through that stage of life.

Shōzen, subscribing to the view first enunciated by Sun Simiao in the mid-seventh century, notes in his introduction to the obstetrics section of the *Ton'ishō* that it was ten times more difficult to treat female ailments than male, since they sprang from more complex causes, and that pregnancy was of the greatest importance to women.[43] In the *Man'anpō* he expresses frustration that, even though he had devoted a chapter to morning sickness (the "child illness"),[44] a condition that he felt was not limited to the first months of pregnancy,[45] what he had covered amounted to "no more than one drop in the vast ocean, or one hair of all those on nine oxen."[46] Nonetheless, while the area to be studied was vast, the goal was to provide better treatment, and older understandings needed to be evaluated. For example, as to when conception might occur,

> I say that [it is the standard view that] after the menstruation every month, the days when one can [conceive] a child are akin to the fertility of the earth itself. However, it is also the case that there are women who become pregnant as a result of intercourse before menstruation. Know this. Is it that one can get pregnant within six days before menstruation? Before menstruation, on days one, three, and five, then it will be a male fetus. On days two, four, and six, then it will be a female child. The day of menstruation each month is determined by the woman. Prior to the monthly event, know the *yin* and *yang* days ([prior days] one, three, and five are *yang,* and two, four, and six are *yin*).[47]

Or regarding the apparent tendency to withhold medicines from pregnant women because of that state, Shōzen's stance was that not prescribing did greater harm than prescribing. This does not mean that Shōzen ignored the condition of pregnancy when prescribing medicines (for example, he notes in the *Ton'ishō* that one medicine must not be administered to pregnant women),[48] but that he felt a blanket prohibition was not a reasonable approach. He buttressed that view by appeal to the authority of Chinese medicine (and of classical Chinese literature):

> I say that in treating the ailments of pregnant women, there are no proscribed medicines. Illnesses kill people. Poisons are themselves serious. Neither the old texts nor the new texts are concerned about proscribed medicines. Now, in pregnant women there are cold damage [disorders], diarrheas, cramps and stiff shoulders, coughing, apoplexy, beriberi, and other assorted illnesses that compete to arise. Therefore the various texts have set down "multiple medicines" in order to treat them. Sometimes the fetus is dead but the mother is still alive; sometimes two lives are joined

as one. How can one take just one view [that medicines ought not be prescribed] and get rid of the wonderful techniques of the old methods? For treating a pregnant woman's morning sickness, works that are employed in the present age such as the *[Heji]ju fang, Qianjin [fang], Waitai [miyao fang]* [外台秘要方, Secret and Essential Formulas of an Outer Censor, 752], *[Taiping] Shenghui [fang], Sanyin [fang],* etc., employ cassia, pinellia, dried ginger, and the like. One should not guard the tree-stump or carve the boat! [i.e., operate on the basis of wrong-headed assumptions].[49]

Another problem was that existing practices sometimes relied upon treatments that would simply not work (even though they seem to have remained part of popular lore for centuries to come).[50] In commenting on Red-Rooted Sage Ointment 丹参膏, an ointment evidently meant to be applied to the body of a pregnant woman, designed to foster the fetus and make it slippery and smooth in order to facilitate an easy birth, Shōzen notes that "In the present age in Japan, this is employed from the seventh month. In many cases they ignore the admonitions that it is not to be represcribed. In recent times in China they do not employ this [Red-Rooted Sage Ointment]. Simply they use Assisting Birth Powder 救生散. This is wonderfully effective."[51]

Shōzen also comments on the role of physicians in the birth process and on the importance of properly treating the umbilical cord:

I say that with a bamboo knife, cutting the length at six *sun* is the best. As to bathing, the theory that this is done after three days is the best. I have some reservations as to the theory that the umbilical cord is to be cut after the newborn infant's first bath; what I fear is that as a result of the bathing there will be an adverse effect on the infant's blood and qi. With methods for cutting the umbilical cord, one must understand the rationale very well and must be very careful with the cutting; simply one has due respect for doing it carefully and properly.[52]

I say that for the methods for tying the umbilical cord simply, the Japanese custom is that it is done in accord with the opinion of an old woman with much experience. If there are any mistakes, then the fault is returned to the physician. If one is asked about any diseases, then accordingly one administers treatment. Even so, one should know the older theories.[53]

Shōzen also identified a major deficiency in traditional approaches to postpartum care, approaches that seem to have been based on custom rather than any informed medical sense of what would facilitate the recuperation of the mother:

> I say that the custom of Japan is that for seven days and seven nights after birth [the woman] does not sleep. This practice is of long-standing. In sum, men and women, whether giving birth or not giving birth, if they go with no sleep and rest for two or three days, then their body and mind are extremely pressed, their blood and qi vital energy is completely deranged. How much more is it the case when a woman who has gone through the labors of childbirth has no rest and sleep for seven days and nights. How can she get any tranquility and peace? As a result of this, mind and soul are extremely pressed, speech is disordered. The physician is unable to render treatment. He himself says that there are malignant spirits and the attending nurse employs prayers. And after all that, she ends up losing her life. This is something for which we must have pity. The *Qianjin [fang], Shenghui [fang], Waitai miyao, Heji[ju fang]* and other texts all have it that after giving birth absolutely she is to go up to the resting area and lie down (not lying down on her side). I have yet to see one text or one medical work which says she is to raise herself up on her knees (and not stretch out her legs). And the theory that from the first night up through the seventh night one does not sleep is a perverted custom 風俗之邪説. Even though the world employs this custom, how can a physician not rectify it?[54]

Shōzen then goes on to cite the section of the *Hejiju fang* on the topic of methods for postpartum care and safeguarding of women, mentions approaches to treatment for some specific problems (such as dizziness), and notes a number of medicines that are to be administered. He elsewhere gives attention to medicines that alleviate postpartum fatigue:

> I say that after the birth is completed, then take a paper-cloth napkin, steep it in vinegar, then place it on the forehead of the birthing woman as if placing the palm of one's hand, and when it has dried then replenish it. It will also ward off agonies and dizziness for thirty to fifty days after the birth. Further, [one can also] heat a number of small stones, steep them in vinegar, then hearing the vapor, day and night [the woman]

> will not be fatigued. If there is dizziness and fatigue then you should provide Purify the Spirit Powder 清魂散, Black Deity Powder 黒神散, Storax Pill 蘇合香円, or Increased Damage Four Ingredient Decoction 增損四物湯. Then after that you should administer treatment according to the symptoms.[55]

SOME CONCLUDING COMMENTS

The spread of print culture in China, the relative explosion of medical writing beginning in the Northern Song and continuing through the Yuan, and the availability of printed Chinese works in the bibliographically rich environment of Kamakura all made it possible for Kajiwara Shōzen to become familiar with Song-period Chinese medicine. He appears to have had access to a larger number and wider variety of Chinese medical writings than anyone else known to us.

Familiarity with Song writings enabled Shōzen to evaluate practices and understandings in Japanese medicine and to become aware of advances in Chinese medical knowledge. Access also permitted him an enhanced sense of the medical endeavor, which sense would not have been possible to obtain within Japan otherwise. Shōzen's engagement also provides us with a glimpse of how Song medicine appeared from outside China. Yet having made that point, it raises the questions, which are beyond the scope of this project, of how Song medicine was seen contemporaneously within China and whether Shōzen, unconstrained by the social dynamics of medicine in China, might have had a more comprehensive sense than Chinese contemporaries. In any event, there is no doubt that Song Chinese medical knowledge transformed his understanding of medicine.

Chapter 3

A SILK ROAD OF PHARMACEUTICALS AND FORMULAS

This chapter highlights the pharmaceutical aspects of the new knowledge available in the East Asian macroculture and shows how Shōzen was a beneficiary of access to and information about materia medica transported along what I call the Pharmaceutical Silk Road. Five topics are discussed: first, the increasing availability of overseas materia medica; second, the technical challenges faced by Shōzen in trying to understand formulas and materia medica; third, some of the changes in Chinese medicine between the Tang and Song eras and the influence of Islamic medicine on Song medicine; and fourth, the new illness category of disorders of qi and Shōzen's understanding of it. Then, I will provide some examples of Shōzen's use of formulas to illustrate how the preceding elements converged to influence Japanese medicine.

INCREASED AVAILABILITY OF OVERSEAS MATERIA MEDICA

Overseas materia medica reached Japan primarily via a multistage maritime trade network that ultimately linked the east coast of Africa, the Arabian Peninsula, the Persian Gulf, coastal ports of India, ports in Southeast Asia (the region as a whole was referred to as the Nanban or Southern Barbarian region), the trading cities of south China such as Ningbo (Hangzhou) and Mingzhou, and the Ryukyu Islands. Through the early fifteenth century, products arrived primarily in ships operated by Chinese merchants and dispatched from southern Chinese ports. We have occasional references to

Japanese pharmacists making purchasing trips to China, but it seems that Chinese merchants also handled the acquisition overseas of the materia medica.[1] From the early fifteenth century, as a result of trade restrictions imposed by the Ming government, Naha in the Ryukyu kingdom became a major transshipment center. One by-product of these shipping arrangements was that sometimes the end users did not know the actual origins of the trade goods: Both Korean and Chinese officials thought that some items of Southeast Asian origin were products of Japan.[2]

Materia medica is known to have been imported into Japan from at least the mid-eighth century.[3] Most items seem to have come from China and were presumably brought by Chinese, but they also came from elsewhere. Merchants involved in the trade came from as far away as Persia.[4] Imported items appear to have been rare and difficult to replace, and agencies of the imperial government kept very detailed records of their use.[5] It is quite likely that leading Buddhist temples maintained their own supplies, employing them primarily as aromatics for ritual activity rather than as medicinal ingredients (although we might be cautious about drawing too sharp a distinction between these uses in this era).[6] Thus they are mentioned in works produced by Buddhist priests, such as *Kōjishō* 香字抄 (Dictionary of Fragrances), *Kōyōshō* 香要抄 (Essentials of Fragrances), *Kōyakushō* 香薬抄 (Book of Fragrances and Medicines), and *Yakushushō* 薬種抄 (Treatise on Materia Medica)[7]—compiled by the priest Ken'i 兼意 in the mid-twelfth century. But they are also noted in the tenth-century (?) *Honzō wamyō* (Japanese Nomenclature for Materia Medica). We lack useful statistics on the amount and frequency with which these items were imported, but we do gain some sense of what items may have been in demand from the 1052 *Shinsarugaku ki* 新猿楽記 (An Account of New Monkey Music). Among goods traded by a fictional merchant, twenty-three aromatic and medicinal items are listed: aloes, musk, cloves, Chinese spikenard, frankincense, birthwort root, Borneo camphor, white sandalwood, the prepared compound "violet snow," croton, realgar, chebulic myrobalan, betel nut, copper rust, cinnabar, pepper powder, rhinoceros horn, ox bezoar, "chicken-tongue" cloves, cnidium, Burmese rosewood, sappan wood, and safflower rouge.[8]

From the mid-thirteenth century, coincident with the growth of cultural and commercial ties across the East China Sea, we have much more useful information about materia medica. That information suggests that items were now available in much larger amounts and on a regular basis, though supply was sometimes interrupted. For example, in the 1270s and 1280s the Mongol Yuan placed an interdiction on trade with Japan in conjunction with preparations for their invasions of the islands. Ironically, or amusingly, Buddhist monks, who at the request of the Kamakura *bakufu* were preparing ceremonies to ward off and subdue the Mongols, complained that "since in recent years the China Ships have not been coming through, materia medica have been difficult to obtain."[9] But by the late thirteenth century, relatively unfettered trade seems to have resumed, and obtaining imported items in the city of Kamakura was an everyday occurrence. One of Shōzen's more interesting comments, which attests in 1304 to the thriving nature of the tea trade and to the popularity of one special variety of tea, is that Wax Tea 臈茶 (臘茶, 蠟茶) "is an item to be compounded, is a China Good [*karamono*], and one buys it from merchants."[10] And in a 1323 document cataloging all the items (and the equivalent cash prices for them) to be supplied for the thirteenth-year memorial service for the *bakufu* leader Hōjō Sadatoki 北条貞時 (1271–1311), we find that at least twenty-five of the sixty-four required materia medica were overseas items.[11]

Lest one thinks that items would have been available in Kamakura because it was a political center and thus their availability in that city is not representative, other sources suggest that this was not the case. One late Kamakura source, a collection of formulas put together by a priest in Nara, notes that he had received a special supply of poppy capsules, wild Siamese cardamom, and ginseng from the Kyoto court physician Wake Tadakage, and he also lists in his formulas fifteen other overseas items.[12] We get a further sense of the ready availability of items when we move past 1333, when Kamakura was destroyed and was no longer a significant center of consumption.

The most striking example comes from the overseas materia medica mentioned in two wound medicine texts, the *Kinsō ryōjishō* 金瘡療治抄 (On Treating Incised Wounds, 1357) and the *Kihō* 鬼法 (Demon Formulas, 1391). These works, inspired by the need to provide emergency treatment for battle injury, listed only ingredients that were known to be available; in fact, it is likely that warfare created a demand for them. The texts list such overseas materia medica as wild Siamese cardamom, Dragon's Blood, musk, cloves, cassia, Burmese rosewood, white sandalwood, aloes, Chinese licorice, turmeric, ginseng, Borneo camphor tree, fennel, frankincense, costus, fossil bones, tiger bones, chebulic myrobalan, ginger, and croton. Ten of these twenty-one items are not noted in the *Shinsarugaku ki* cited earlier.

Materia medica noted in another fourteenth-century medical work, the *Fukudenpō* 福田方 (Formulas from the Fields of Merit), also attest to the availability of overseas items.[13] Twenty-eight of the 114 materia medica noted in the *Fukudenpō* are Song additions to the Chinese pharmacopoeia. At the risk of repetition, these are Chinese clematis, corydalis, poppy capsule, pagoda tree, *chianghuo,* greater galangal, rice sprout, black pepper, fenugreek, Siberian moonseed, persimmon, immature orange, pokeroot, *tsaoko,* Chinese honey locust, mulberry, Katsumada's galangal (round cardamom), betel seed, bamboo juice and bamboo shavings, matrimony vine, cardamom, rice paper, barley sprouts, arsenic, fushen, borax, and Chinese myrica.[14] Items in the *Fukudenpō* are also of interest because the additions to the Chinese pharmacopoeia included items originating from Southeast Asia, South Asia, Southwest Asia, and the Middle East. The items include aloeswood, cloves, *agastache,* costus, mandarin orange, immature orange, lesser galangal, ginger, *tsaoko,* Katsumada's galangal, cardamom, grains of paradise, *ichihjen, zedoary,* black pepper, nutmeg, greater galangal, cassia, asafoetida, Sumatra benzoin, frankincense, betel nut, chebulic myrobalan, and Dragon's Blood.[15]

In short, in the fourteenth century a wide variety of overseas materia medica was readily available. It goes without saying that the formulas listed in the *Ton'ishō* and the *Man'anpō* were working formulas and not ones noted merely for reference. However, while materia medica was increasingly available, that availability presented its own problems.

UNDERSTANDING MATERIA MEDICA: THE TECHNICAL CHALLENGES

The increased amount and variety of overseas materia medica available in Japan from the late thirteenth century enabled physicians to compound and prescribe the thousands of new formulas noted in Song medical works. Using their standard tools—mortars, pestles, cups, spoons, medicine grinders, flat-dish scales with counterweights, and paper packets for the medicinal materials—they were able to prepare ingredients and medicines with facility.[16] In order to prepare medicines, however, Shōzen and others had to confront some technical issues, which required them to be technical translators as well as technological transmitters. For our purposes, there were three main technical challenges. The first was to understand correctly dosage and measurement. The second involved the proper identification of materia medica, the correcting of earlier misidentifications, and ensuring that formula names were appropriate. The third was the issue of substitution when ingredients were unavailable.

Measurements and Dosages

In premodern Japan and perhaps throughout East Asia, standards for weights and measurements were neither unchanging nor uniform. Even though units of measurement might remain the same, the metrics of a given unit might vary from place to place and time to time. Chinese dynasties—the Tang and the Song, for example—introduced new standards in order to rectify inconsistencies and in the process also establish their authority and legitimacy. However, these efforts might also cumulatively add to the problem, since formulas themselves did not provide information on the standards of measurement used in that formula. For Japanese physicians who engaged Chinese formulas, this was a constant problem over the centuries (and continued after Shōzen's day).[17] Thus we find a section in Renki's *Chōsei ryōyōhō* (Formulas for Fostering Long Life) devoted to various measurement standards and equivalences. He carefully explains the measuring standards appearing in the *Bencaojing* 本草経 (Classic of Materia Medica) and also alludes to varying standards of measurement within Japan.[18] Yet it is evident that, writing in the 1180s, Renki was unaware of the restandardizations that had taken place after the Song reunified China two centuries earlier.

When Shōzen became aware that there were new standards, he had no prior guidelines to help him understand those standards. He thus had to correlate earlier measurement standards with the new Song ones, in addition to confirming what standards were in use in the over twenty thousand formulas contained in the printed medical works that he was assessing. Here and there he draws attention to the issue, as when he notes that "With this medicine, apart from the jujube, it should be twenty-two *ryō* 両. The reason for this is that in the Tang Zhengyao era the Tang court made four *seni* 銭 equivalent to one *ryō,*" and he then goes on to make calculations for other measurements as well.[19] Elsewhere we encounter different equivalences for *seni* and *ryō:* "eight, nine *ryō* are four *seni,* one *ryō* is (comprised of) eighty pills *gan* 丸, so is it that nine *ryō* is thus eight nines seventy-two seven hundred and twenty pills?"[20] Shōzen may not have had to make calculations for every single formula, but the process seems to have been both frequent and frustrating:[21]

> I say that with regard to what is a little amount of musk and frankincense, the *Youyou xinshu* states that one *bu* 分 is insufficient, and I call this a small amount. This is within one to two *seni* or three to four *seni.* Root of common achyranthes denotes local achyranthes grown in the wild. Fruit of common puncture-vine, common Chinese allspice, and common fennel are all likewise [grown in the wild]. For one *gō* 合 the *Bencao* [Pharmocopoeia] gauging for *shō* 升 and *gō* notes that "for *shō* the rule is that the top diameter is one *sun* 寸, the bottom diameter six *bu,* and the depth is eight *bu.*" This is a *gō.* With this *gō,* ten *gō* constitute one *shō.* However, this is the Tang court's *shō.* The Song court's *shō* takes three of the old *gō* and makes it now one *gō* and takes three of the old *shō* and makes it now one *shō.* (These are the explanations from the *Sanyin fang* and the *Youyou xinshu*). Consequently now as to one *gō* of bidentate achyranthes, this *Bencao*'s three *gō* constitute one [current] *gō.* Further the *Sanyin [fang]* says that "one large *sakazuki* 盞 patterns on one *shō,* and one medium *sakazuki* patterns on five *gō,* one small *sakazuki* patterns on three *gō.*" Here too the *Bencao*'s three *gō* constitute one *gō,* and ten *gō* constitute one large *sakazuki,* etc. I Shōzen have a one-volume work *Shōgōron* 升合論 [Discourse on Shō and Gō] that one should look at. One cannot memorize all this.

I find it difficult to disagree with this final assessment.

Another concern was determining appropriate dosage, a task that involved two elements. The first element involved clarifying whether the doses for the same formula found in different sources were the same or not, determining how the doses would be calculated, and deciding what adjustments might be necessary in using them. For example, when dealing with a formula for treating pelvic pain caused by movement of the fetus between the second and third to eighth and ninth months, Shōzen notes that "one dose of the old formula is strong," so he makes adjustments based on the new formula.[22] In another example, he notes that "In the old formula [for Storax Pill 蘇合香丸], one pill is prescribed, but in the newly arrived *[Furen] Daquan liangfang,* four pills are prescribed.[23] The second element involved making adjustments to the original formula based on clinical experience so that the prescriptions would be optimal. We encounter many such references, and Shōzen usually refers to himself in the first person. For example, instead of ten pills per dose, he notes that it should be thirty to fifty pills, or in a recipe that calls for forty granules, he notes that the dose should be a hundred granules.[24] On other occasions, his comment is more extensive: For Realgar Pill 雄黄丸 (used for treating chronic indigestion and dyspepsia), he notes that the amount of the dosage is too small and does not have efficacy, one must give double the amount, and it must normally be used at the rate of one dose every two or three days.[25]

Identification, Recognition, Naming

The second technical challenge involved terminology for materia medica. First, there appears to have been some confusion over accurate identification caused by such factors as the lack of a uniform authority record for terminology and the use of many local names for botanicals. Second, earlier Japanese reference works sometimes misidentified items, mistakes that only became apparent with access to newer materials.

These problems were well known in late-thirteenth-century Japan. The court physician Koremune Tomotoshi noted that people, himself included, failed to recognize specialized use of Chinese characters or the use of variant names.[26] Tomotoshi was sufficiently concerned that by 1284 he had compiled the *Honzō iroha shō* (Materia Medica in Japanese Alphabetical Order), an in-depth reference guide to variant vocabulary and terminology appearing in the Chinese *Daguan bencao* (Daguan Era Materia Medica, 1108). However, as we have earlier noted, while the *Honzō iroha shō* and its extensive cross-referencing was the first Japanese work in over a century to address issues of identification, it was unavailable to Shōzen. Accordingly, Shōzen had to produce his own reference material.

Shōzen first addressed the terminology issue in the *Ton'ishō,*[27] but his most extensive treatment appears in two essays—the *Yakumei ruijū* 薬名類聚 (Collation of Materia Medica Terminology) and the *Shōmi kagami* 賞味鏡 (Mirror That Illuminates Flavors)—that he wrote between the completion of the *Man'anpō* in 1327 and 1331 (these later became the final four chapters of the *Man'anpō*).[28] The *Yakumei ruijū* is roughly 295 pages in length and has at least 2,200 entries for names of materia medica. Though the information provided on each varies, it includes such things as the flavor of a drug, whether it might be a "hot" or a "cold" item, the Japanese pronunciation of the Chinese characters for a name, sometimes a variant Japanese name for the item, and whether it is a variant name for something else. Sometimes he makes his own identification, such as "I say that this is a *mukade* centipede."[29]

The *Shōmi kagami* is roughly 246 pages in length and provides more fulsome information on approximately 130 minerals, plants, trees, four-legged animals, birds, fish, bivalves, fruit, nuts, grains, flavorings, and suchlike. The most complete entries list both Chinese and Japanese names, but some have only Chinese ones. The information is taken overwhelmingly from Chinese sources. The source reference is usually noted, and not infrequently more than one source is used. The descriptions are lengthy, and the afflictions for which the materia medica is suitable are noted. On occasion Shōzen adds his own remarks, which include comparisons of new information with that in Fukane Sukebito's tenth-century *Honzō wamyō.*[30]

What are some of the issues addressed in these two works? One issue was vocabulary, which entailed clarifying differences in Chinese and Japanese vocabulary or providing the colloquial Japanese name to which the Chinese characters referred. The most obvious way of doing this was to place Japanese readings next to Chinese characters for materia medica and items, as we find for example in lists of permitted and prohibited foods.[31] In some cases a common Japanese term was applied to a range of Chinese terms. For example, the term "abalone sore" was applied to "sore circly"; to the reversed term "circly sore"; and the "rashy-palm sore" could be equated to "insect sore," "abalone sore," or "sore with an insect in it."[32] We also find that "Carpesium" is referred to in Chinese as "crane lice" but in Japanese as "dog's bum."[33] In other cases, Shōzen notes points of interest; for example, whereas a Chinese text will refer to "tortoise chest," the *Wamyō* [*Honzō wamyō*] notes that the Japanese equivalent is "pigeon chest."[34]

A second issue was the identification of information, which entailed noting mistakes and clarifying differences between Chinese and Japanese varieties of an item. At some point Shōzen realized that he could not take existing Japanese identifications of materia medica for granted and would need to rectify the errors. He does not mention how much time he spent doing this, to what extent he benefited from Chinese informants, or whether the identifications were systematic or serendipitous. However, one senses that Shōzen, like the precise compiler of the *Honzō irohashō,* confirmed every item.

Among the errors that he found in the old reference work *Honzō wamyō* were such misidentifications as chrysanthemum as mugwort, sheat fish as sweetfish, grass carp as mackerel, clam as paddy shell, bitter orange as citron, chestnut as filbert, or salmon as perch.[35] In other cases he notes common errors, such as equating the seed of the opium poppy with the seed of white mustard or thinking that mercury was yellow ochre.[36] We do not know how much time it took Shōzen to identify and correct an error, but in some instances we get the sense it might occupy him for an extended period. One such example involved ascertaining the difference between eel and moray eel, which, as becomes clear, he seems to have been unable to resolve satisfactorily. Shōzen remarks in one place that the eel *(shiriuo, Anguilla japonica)* is a large version of the *tsuchikujiri* and is a proven medicine for debilitation associated with corpse-transmitted diseases. In other places he notes that moray eel *(utsubuuo, Monopterus albus)* is eel *(unagi)*; that the *Honzō wamyō* equates this moray eel *(utsubuuo)* with bent old lady *(kome)* or lobster *(ebi, Panulirus japonicus)*, which is not correct; and that regarding the term for eel *(shiriuo)*, the *Honzō wamyō* identifies it as *hajikamiiwo*, another theory suggests that it is eel *(unagi)*, and he himself identifies it as *tsuchikujiri*.[37]

A related area of identification was determining if Chinese and Japanese varieties were sufficiently different as to require adjustments to formulas. For example, in the case of the cinnabar ingredient in the *Hejiju fang* formula for Divine Transcendant's Fundamental Ointment 神仙太一膏, Shōzen notes that the method of preparation and amount of ingredient used will vary depending on whether one employs Chinese cinnabar or Japanese cinnabar.[38] He also discovered that the granules for croton and apricot came in small and large varieties, and that there were differences between the Chinese and the Japanese ones.[39] And in numerous places he notes that formulas that use jujubes will have to be adjusted since Japanese jujubes are smaller than Chinese ones.[40]

A final concern related to terminology was the names of formulas. As a rule of thumb, the names of Chinese formulas were adopted without change. The Chinese characters remained the same, and in speech, as was customary, the Japanese pronunciation was applied to the title. On rare occasions, however, it appears that the Japanese pronunciation was infelicitous, and that an alternate name was desirable. A good example is provided by the medicine Purple Pill 紫円 (Ch. Ziyuan, Ja. Shien), which was used for treating infant febrile ailments. When Shōzen noted it in the *Ton'ishō*, he remarked simply that it was an alternate name (along with Purple Prime Pill 紫元子, Shigenshi) for Purple Frost Pill 紫霜円

(Shisōen).[41] Later, however, there seems to have been some concern that the Japanese pronunciation of Purple Pill was a homophone for Death Pill 死円 (Ch. Siyuan, Ja. Shien), hardly an encouraging name when treating infants (or anyone else, for that matter). Accordingly, in the *Man'anpō* Shōzen renamed it: "I name this and call it Cinnabar Prime Pill 丹元子 (Tangenshi), the reason being that the violet 紫 (*shi*) and death 死 (*shi*) characters are homophones and are normally avoided."[42]

Availability and Substitution

The third technical issue confronting users of overseas materia medica was availability. Availability of ingredients was not confined to overseas items, of course, and as noted earlier, in general overseas items were readily available. However, if a particular item was not immediately to hand or was perhaps difficult to get, then people needed to think of alternatives. When there was uncertainty over the correspondence between apparently similar Japanese and Chinese varieties of an item, authors were adamant that only the indicated Chinese item should be used, and no alternative was considered.[43] But on other occasions, alternatives were recommended as a matter of course.

In some cases the issue that presented itself was whether the physician should use a formula at all, as some ingredients were difficult to obtain. Answers varied. If only one item (ox gallstone) was difficult to obtain but other items (centipede, rock lizard, and Chinese blister fly) were easy to get, then the formula was worth using.[44] When all the ingredients (ox gallstone, Tiger's eye [literally], brain musk [脳麝, unidentified], and scorpion) were difficult to obtain, then the formula was not recommended.[45] In other cases, alternative formulas were recommended.[46]

In other instances the question became what substitutes would be used. Amber, though listed in a Chinese source as existing in Japan, does not seem to have been indigenous.[47] It was, however, important in formulas for such complaints as sudden swelling of the lower abdomen or choleric dysentery as a result of a change in the position of the fetus (Amber Decoction 琥珀湯), lack of menstrual flow (Soft-Shell Tortoise Shell Pill 鱉甲丸), and where an infant may have a bleeding cut or a sore abdomen as a result of being dropped on the floor or having fallen on the ground (Cattail Powder 蒲黄散).[48] Shōzen felt that Japanese Frankincense 日本薫陸 was a good substitute.[49] In another example, the domestic items mulberry white-bark and silkworm dung could be employed as substitutes for the hard-to-obtain overseas item, praying mantis egg case, found on a mulberry branch.[50] In some cases, the substitute was also an overseas item: If clematis was unavailable, then Chinese licorice or Cape jasmine fruit could be used;[51] if seed of abutilon was unavailable, then one used yellow hollyhock.[52]

In sum, absorbing the overseas materia medica was not a seamless process. It required technical translation, scientific inquiry, and extensive clinical evaluation. Employing the wider range of materia medica also meant that a new pharmaceutical regime was being adopted.

EVOLVING CHINESE FORMULAS AND ISLAMIC MEDICINE

There were substantial changes in the Chinese pharmaceutical regime from the Tang through the Song dynasties. These changes had a direct influence on medieval Japanese medicine, and they are embodied in Shōzen's texts. Among the developments, we note a greater use of nondecoction medicines such as powders and pills, the increased complexity of formulas, and a greater variety of materia medica. These developments are generally well known. Less well known is that the changes were also influenced by formulas and materia medica that derived from Islamic medicine. I will look first at some broader changes and then at the Islamic influence.

The first topic emerges clearly when we look at the changes in Japanese context by comparing formulas from the *Ishinpō,* which is based on Tang medicine, and from the *Man'anpō,* which is based on Song medicine. Since both works are voluminous, I will take an example from one area—children's medicine—to illustrate the changes.

The fact that there are 462 formulas related to pediatrics in the *Ishinpō* and 1,121 in the eleven chapters of the pediatrics section of the *Man'anpō* (which draws heavily from the *Youyou xinshu*)[53] already highlights one major development from Tang to Song: Namely, there was simply a great deal more medical activity. Beyond number, however, it is the actual composition of the formulas that is of interest here. A comparison reveals three main changes. First, there is a pronounced shift from using medicines that are externally applied to medicines that are internally administered. Whereas in the *Ishinpō* 61 percent (281) of the formulas are for external application and 36 percent (168) for internal application, in the *Man'anpō* the ratios are more than reversed, 24 percent (271) and

67 percent (756) respectively. Second, with respect to internally administered medicines, there is a pronounced shift away from a preponderant use of decoction medicines to the use of a wider range of forms. Whereas in the *Ishinpō* virtually all of the internally administered medicines are decoctions, in the *Man'anpō* they account for only 40 percent (304) of the formulas. The other 60 percent (452) came in forms that were only rarely used prior to the Song—namely powders, granules, and pills.[54]

The third noteworthy change was that formulas became more complex. There was a pronounced shift away from formulas comprised of only one or two ingredients (92 percent in the *Ishinpō* versus 47 percent in the *Man'anpō*) to formulas containing three (4 percent versus 11 percent) or, far more common, four or more ingredients (3 percent versus 42 percent). Note too that while the ratios changed, the total number of single-ingredient formulas remained fairly constant (339 versus 362). The single-ingredient formulas in the *Man'anpō* derive almost exclusively from earlier works regarded in the Song as classics, such as the *Shanghan lun* (On Cold Damage Disorders) or the *Qianjin fang* (Priceless Formulas). This suggests perhaps that the broader changes did not connote a wholesale replacement of earlier formulas but included a winnowing process that identified which earlier formulas were effective and augmented and expanded the knowledge base with newer formulas. This raises the question of what may have contributed to the increasing complexity of formulas.

The second topic is the influence of Islamic (Arabic) medicine on Song Chinese medicine. Recent research, focusing on a comparison of the *Hejiju fang* with earlier Chinese works, has shown conclusively that Song medicine incorporated materia medica and approaches to complex, multi-ingredient formulas that are found in Islamic medicine but that are not attested in pre-Song Chinese pharmaceutical traditions. The research has also found that while Islamic medicine had a demonstrable impact overall, the impact varied from area to area. For example, whereas Islamic medicine had only a small impact in the area of treatments for cold damage disorders (exogenous febrile diseases),[55] it had a significant influence on formulas used to treat a category of disorders that was itself new in the Song, "all forms of [disorders of] qi," and the influence is particularly noticeable in formulas for aromatic stomachics.[56] I will thus look at these formulas.

Pre-Tang Chinese medical literature contains very few formulas for aromatic stomachics. In contrast, their use is highly developed in Islamic medicine, and as seen in Ibn-Sīnā's classic *Canon of Medicine,* those formulas have three distinct characteristics. First, there are large numbers of materia medica compounded in any one formula: In the *Canon,* over half of the formulas contain over fifteen drugs, while one of them has as many as sixty-four drugs. Second, while many materia medica may be included in a formula, many of them have similar medicinal qualities. Third, the most frequently used materia medica include ginger, cardamoms, peppers, botanicals from the Umbelliferae family (such as angelica, coriander, cumin, fennel, asafoetida, and lovage), items in the camphor family such as cinnamon bark, and tannin items such as chebulic myrobalan.

Formulas reflecting these various characteristics are common in the *Hejiju fang.* This does not reflect developments internal to Chinese medicine but influences from Islamic medicine. This emerges clearly from a comparison of formulas found in the 752 *Waitai miyao fang* (Secret and Essential Formulas of an Outer Censor) and in the early Northern Song *Taiping Shenghui fang,* with the 108 formulas in the "all forms of [disorders of] qi" section of the *Hejiju fang.* Within the formulas, two elements are central to the comparisons: the number of materia medica in the aromatic and the salty categories and which of these are of traditional Chinese origin and which ones are of Western origin (a term broadly indicating the modern Middle East, Southwest Asia, South Asia, and perhaps Southeast Asia). Some detail is required to explicate the argument, but I will keep it to a minimum.

Three points emerge from the comparison. First, of the fifty aromatic or salty items in the *Hejiju fang,* twenty-nine (60 percent) are of Western origin; only four of these twenty-nine are noted in the *Waitai miyao fang* (lesser galangal, birthwort root, cardamom, and black pepper); nineteen are cited in the *Taiping Shenghui fang.* Second, there is little difference in the listing of traditional Chinese aromatics and spices between the *Waitai miyao* and the *Hejiju fang,* suggesting that the Western-origin drugs augmented rather than supplanted Chinese ones.[57] Third, in earlier Chinese medicine, few aromatics and fewer spicy aromatics were used, but they enjoyed a high rate of usage because one or two were generally included in a formula. By contrast, the formulas in the *Hejiju fang* reflect the characteristics of those in Ibn-Sīnā's *Canon of Medicine.* In the *Canon,* a large number of aromatics and spicy medicinals are employed, though the rate of usage of any one is comparatively low since many were compounded together.

That there was a substantial change in the usage of Western-origin materia medica in the four hundred years between the compilation of the

Waitai miyao fang and that of the *Hejiju fang* might not occasion surprise. However, there was also a significant change in the roughly 150 years between the *Taiping shenghui fang* of 992 and the *Hejiju fang* of 1151.[58] Looking at the Western-origin materia medica in the *Hejiju fang,* I note ten new materia medica (nut grass, clove peel, spikenard, sandalwood, turmeric, Sumatra benzoin, storax, frankincense, birthwort root,[59] and myrrh), a dramatic increase in the use of six items previously known (grains of paradise, *zedoary,* aloeswood, *agastache*, fennel, and black pepper), and a notable increase in the use of another six known items (musk, *ichihjen,* cardamom, nutmeg, lesser galangal, and cloves), and there is a slight drop in the use of costus root. Another six items are common to both works but do not appear in the *Waitai miyao* (*tsaoko,* cubebs, another term for frankincense, asafoetida, long pepper, and Borneo camphor). The reader may observe that there is considerable overlap between these materia medica and ones noted earlier as being available in Japan.

To summarize this discussion, there were some significant developments in Chinese pharmacology from Tang through Song. Some of those developments were propelled by knowledge of materia medica and compounding protocols derived from Islamic medicine. One notable area of influence was in a new category, the "all forms of [disorders of] qi."

DISORDERS OF QI 気 AND ISLAMIC MEDICINE IN JAPAN

Disorders of Qi

The illness category of "all forms of [disorders of] qi" first appeared in Chinese medical writing in the *Hejiju fang,* and along with the Western-origin materia medica in the formulas in the category it was widely employed thereafter.[60] As we know, the *Hejiju fang* was extensively used by Shōzen. As noted earlier, it was the second-largest source of formulas in the *Ton'ishō* (providing 220, after the 258 from the *Taiping Shenghui fang*), and the third-largest source of formulas in the *Man'anpō* (providing 156, after the 217 from the *Taiping Shenghui fang* and the 1,797 from the *Shengji zonglu*). Naturally enough, Shōzen learned about this new category of "all forms of [disorders of] qi" as a result of reading the *Hejiju fang,* and he regarded it as a significant new category. Revealingly, of the 155 or so formulas included in the *Ton'ishō* and the *Man'anpō* that apply to "all forms of [disorders of] qi," only about 20 percent of them (thirty-two) are drawn from the *Hejiju fang* itself. Even more remarkable is that seventy-seven formulas (almost 50 percent of the total) are taken from the the *Shengji zonglu,* which does not even *have* the ailment category of "all forms of [disorders of] qi." (The remaining 30 percent include twelve from the *Keyong fang* and ten from the *Yuyaoyuan fang.*)

Shōzen had clearly spent time choosing formulas for this new category, so the obvious question is: Why? As far as I can tell, Shōzen was not aware of the influence of Islamic medicine on Chinese medicine (the *Hejiju fang* itself provides no explicit information), so this would not have been a reason. And, while positive clinical experience with the formulas would obviously be a factor, clinical success does not explain why the formulas would have been used in the first place (one may of course assume that he would have been interested in trying something new). However, one reason the category appealed to him seems to be that the nosology of the category confirmed some fundamental Buddhist understandings on the causes of illness—particularly the perception that states of mind lie behind illness.

Medieval Japanese sources make it clear that it was generally understood that states of mind (emotions) could have an influence on behavior and that this could be manifested in physical symptoms.[61] These emotions cover a familiar range—such as madness, grief, depression, love sickness, and aberrant behavior—that seems to derive from some disorder of the mind. At least one medical text denotes cowardice as a state of mind that can be manifested in physical symptoms: "There are those who are afraid and lose their ability to speak either on the battlefield or in the presence of the elevated. It is said that there are those, usually inferiors, who on such occasions vomit blood."[62] More prosaically, but perhaps reflecting general common sense about mind and symptoms, the disciples of the noted Zen priest Ikkyū (1398–1481) believed that his attacks of diarrhea were directly related to and triggered by his moods.[63] All of these emotions could be understood in terms of imbalance of qi.

Shōzen addresses qi in three chapters in the *Ton'ishō* (chapters 10, 11, and 12) and in one chapter of the *Man'anpō* (25). While he has numerous remarks about it in these chapters, for our purposes his most salient comments appear in chapter 12 of the *Ton'ishō.*[64] In the preface to the chapter, Shōzen makes clear that the category of "all forms of [disorders of] qi" refers to illnesses produced by what is understood as "internal causes," as explicated in the *Sanyin fang.* However, when explicating broader understandings of disease causation noted in the *Sanyin fang,* Shōzen himself introduces perspectives that are independent of and additional to what we find in the *Sanying fang.* He correlates the idea of illness originating from internal causes with an understanding regarding the cause of illness that is basic to Buddhism.

In chapter 12, Shōzen begins by mentioning that there is a Tian heaven yin and yang that correlates with three yin and three yang in humans, and that there are five elements in the earth that correlate with the five viscera (heart, lungs, liver, spleen, kidneys) and five bowels (small intestine, colon, gallbladder, stomach, and bladder) in humans.[65] There are also 404 ailments, as well as the 10,000 myriad illnesses. In trying to understand all these, Chao Yuan[fang] 巢元方 in his *[Zhu]bing yuanhou [zong]lun* 諸病源候總論 (General Treatise on the Etiology and Symptomology of Diseases) designated 1,800 categories under which he subsumed and explained all ailments. However, as even this schemata proved inadequate for explaining the 10,000 myriad illnesses, later Chen Yan 陳言 in his *Sanyin fang* categorized the 10,000 myriad illnesses into three categories of causes. These three categories were internal causes, external causes, and causes neither internal nor external.

Shōzen then goes on to explicate the causes. His explanations for the external causes category and of causes neither internal nor external follow the explanations in the *Sanyin fang.* External causes are ailments produced when the six objects external to the body (wind, cold, summer heat, dampness, dryness, and heat) come and damage people's skin and, without particular cause, produce ailments. Causes that are neither internal nor external include such things as starvation, overeating, being gnawed by a tiger, being bitten by an insect, being wounded by a blade, muscles and bones being struck or broken, being hit by a rock, drowning in water, damaging muscle and bone through falling from a carriage horse or high place, being burned by a flame, or being scalded by hot water. These injuries are not to be confused with problems caused by external causes, and likewise they do not come from anything internal to the body.

When addressing internal causes, however, Shōzen introduces perspectives that are independent of information in the *Sanyin fang.* As noted, he correlates the idea that illness may arise from internal causes with understandings of illness causation that are fundamental to Buddhism. Shōzen starts off by noting, as does the *Sanyin fang,* that internal causes are found where illnesses are produced from the disorder of the seven qi vital energies of joy, anger, melancholy, worry, sadness, fear, and fright. To illustrate how emotions can cause illness, Shōzen then recounts the well-known Chinese story of Yueguang 楽廣, who exhibited severe symptoms and became ill because he had imagined that he had swallowed a snake.[66] What had in fact happened is that he mistook the reflection of a bow in his wine for a snake and thought that he had drunk the snake.

Having established that some problems arise in the mind (*kokoro, xin,* 心), Shōzen then proceeds to argue that in such cases the mind needs to be treated. He draws a parallel with an analogy that he attributes to the *Avatamsaka Sutra* 華厳経 (Flower Ornament Sutra). Since Shōzen rarely refers to any Buddhist texts by name, it is clear that he wants to make a profound rather than a casual point. He makes the point that when treating ailments of the mind, one must treat the mind: The analogy he adduces is that of a teacher of wisdom who, in order to make the point that delusion and comprehension both reside in the mind but are two sides of the same thing, alternately displays the back and the palm of the hand to illustrate that they are both components of the hand. He then makes his main point that the *Avatamsaka Sutra*'s teaching is that the ailments of the three poisons (greed, anger, and delusion) of evil passions arise from the mind. Accordingly, all of the afflictions that arise from the imbalance of the seven qi arise from the mind. Once someone realizes this point, then emotions are neither produced nor activated, the blood and qi are harmonized, and the mind and the body are at rest.

To sum this up, Shōzen agrees that the phrase "all forms of [disorders of] qi" indicates illnesses from internal causes. Such illnesses are understood in Chinese ideas as being caused by disorders of the qi and that those disorders are caused by delusion. This, then, means that the Chinese ideas accord with the Buddhist notion that delusion arises from the mind and that to treat the delusions, one must then treat the mind.

As a clinical physician, Shōzen primarily treated the body. However, it is clear that because of the fact that in treating illnesses of the qi one would be engaging in the fundamental act of Buddhist healing, he also worked to heal illnesses of the mind. Accordingly, the new illness category would be considered a very profound one and worth adopting. The obvious corollary is that the formulas that fall into that category—and of course the ingredients that are used in the formula—would be highly regarded.

Shōzen's Comments on Formulas

I conclude with some examples showing how Shōzen evaluated these new formulas that reflected the influences of Islamic medicine on Chinese medicine and thus indirectly influenced medieval Japanese medicine. I could of course simply note that the hundreds of formulas in *Ton'ishō* and *Man'anpō* that use overseas materia medica and that contain multiple ingredients (as many as thirty-three in one case) leave no doubt about the matter. However, Shōzen's responses convey a sense of the excitement for the new medicines that a cataloging cannot. Following are some comments on a formula that treats "all forms of [disorders of] qi," a formula that was based on storax, and some formulas created by Shōzen.

The first example suggests not only that Shōzen actively embraced the new category of "all forms of [disorders] of qi" but that he seems to have come to the conclusion that qi itself was an important nosology and that formulas for specific ailments might have wider application. The formula, Coiling Leek Powder 蟠葱散, was taken from the *Hejiju fang*. It was prescribed for a variety of ailments that affected males, females, and pregnant women, such as lack of appetite, regurgitation, heatstroke, leukorrheal discharges, and prepartum and postpartum chills, fevers, and abdominal pains. It was composed of twelve ingredients, six of Chinese origin (Chinese atractylodes, licorice, bur reed, immature orange, poria, and corydalis) and six of Western origin (*zedoary*, cardamom, cloves, betel palm, cinnamon, and dried ginger).

> This is a wonderful medicine for treating "all forms of [disorders of] qi," and one cannot write enough about it. It is explained and discussed in various works. The hundred ailments arise from the qi. But medicines that readjust the qi thereby treat the myriad illnesses and can't go wrong. The *Sanyin fang* takes the seven qi illnesses and considers them to be illnesses from internal causes. It takes summer heat wetness syndrome caused by wind evil, relapse of illness caused by overconsumption, and considers them illnesses from external causes. It takes hot water, fire, arrow, and blade injuries and considers them illnesses from neither internal nor external causes. Consequently those arising from within and from the mind [心] are considered internal causes. Most certainly [this formula] accords with this reasoning. One must certainly be grateful for the various works and formulas.[67]

The second example is the aromatic stomachic Storax Pill 蘇合香圓. This formula appears to have been well known in Shōzen's day. In fact, a contemporary resident of Kamakura, the Chinese physician Zhiguang, enjoyed a reputation as a compounder of medicines and in particular as a provider of the Storax Pill.[68] There are two notable aspects to Storax Pill. The first is that of the sixteen possible materia medica in the formula, fourteen were of Western origin (storax, frankincense, Borneo camphor, white sandalwood, cloves, cinnabar, nutgrass, rhinoceros horn, musk, Sumatra benzoin, long pepper, chebulic myrobalan, aloeswood, costus). Second, there were a number of versions of it (Shōzen lists five), which seems to suggest that, even while the variations were minor, it was widely used and physicians made adjustments to it as a result of their own experimentation or, possibly, the availability of the ingredients.[69]

Shōzen too made his own adjustments and suggestions on what he described as wonder medicine 神薬.[70] For example, in one case he suggested that whereas the formula in the *Shengji zonglu* directed that the dose should be ten pills (three pills for old people and children), on an empty stomach and washed down with well water, he remarked that the dose should be thirty to fifty pills.[71] In another case he noted that as an alternative to using Perellia Syrup 紫蘇飲, one should administer Storax Pill or Rectify Qi Powder 正気散 and increase their effectiveness by adding *burpleurum* or ginger.[72] In another place, he was quite effusive:

> I say that this medicine is the absolute best for suffering associated with all kinds of rising of qi and irritability. Therefore it is explained clearly at the beginning of this chapter. For infant measles, exogenous febrile diseases and diseases due to summer heat, and those of internal heat and dryness heat syndrome, in all cases one should administer cold water. If the body is cold and fatigued, then one should warm up the medicine with heat and have it prepared as a warm decoction. Or else administer it along with warm rice wine. This is the lore of Storax Pill. One must be extremely grateful for this.[73]

A third example of Shōzen's engagement is that he came up with formulas of his own. This was unusual. As far as I have been able to discover, while Shōzen compared formulas and made adjustments and on occasion renamed a formula, he developed only two of his own.[74] The first formula was a by-product of his use of Storax Pill. He notes that not only was it "marvelously efficacious" to double the amounts of Borneo camphor, musk, and cinnabar, one could omit Borneo camphor and increase the amount of musk and rename the formula Musk Storax 麝香蘇, which was marvelous for treating people suffering from cold of deficiency type and from intestinal worms.[75] The second formula that Shōzen designed was for treating diarrhea.

Diarrhea and enteric ailments generally, particularly in the summer months, were a perennial concern of physicians in the medieval era (and no doubt other periods as well).[76] What stands out in Shōzen's work is that the most efficacious formulas are ones that rely upon Western-origin materia medica, which of course means that this is another area where we can identify the impact of new materia medica. One of the formulas, Ox Gallstone Agada Pill 牛黄阿伽陀円, which may have been an Indian Buddhist formula, was comprised of fifteen ingredients, eight of which were of Western origin.[77] The formula was regarded highly: "As to the method of compounding, one must receive the oral transmission. This is not to be transmitted casually. The oral transmission is written down separately; it is the most secret of the secret."[78] Another formula, Nutmeg Powder 肉豆蔻散, three of whose four ingredients were of Western origin, also seems to have been a powerful weapon in the medical arsenal. Shōzen remarks that it is to be used for treating all types of red and white diarrhea, when other medicines have no efficacy and there is no end to the shitting.[79] Against this background, Shōzen developed his own Hundred Centered Powder 百中散 comprised of the Western-origin ingredients nutmeg, cardamom, and cloves. Claiming that his Hundred Centered Powder is 100 percent effective for all diarrheas, he instructs as follows:

> Grind the ingredients, each dose to be five to seven *seni* or six to seven *seni.* It is to be administered on an empty stomach before meals, either with rice gruel or chestnut gruel; three to four doses per day, or at the very least two to three doses; this is guaranteed to work. If the diarrhea has stopped then you can administer Grain Esteemed Powder 禾嘉散[80] or Six Flavor Eight Flavor Calming Stomach Powder 六味八味平胃散; if there is still a little diarrhea then to Grain Esteemed Powder or Calming Stomach Powder add two to three *seni* of nutmeg and administer that, then the person will be cured. This is to be used for high and low, old and young, adults and children.[81]

SOME CONCLUDING COMMENTS

It is clear that from the Kamakura period, Japan was the beneficiary of a great deal of new knowledge about formulas and materia medica that was able to be put to clinical use because of expanded access to a wide range of materia medica that were, most immediately, available in China. We have also seen that the Chinese pharmaceutical regime was in turn the beneficiary of information and items that originated from areas throughout Asia and the Middle East. From the Song onwards, there were noticeable advances in the complexity of medicines, in the form of the medicines, and in the variety of materia medica employed. One of the notable aspects of these changes was the influence of Arabic or Islamic medicine on Chinese medicine.

However, integrating that knowledge entailed a substantial amount of what we may call technical translation. One of the issues was trying to clarify and regularize varying standards of measurement. Shōzen also had to identify some of the materia medica listed in formulas, as well as rectifying mistaken identifications that had been made in earlier Japanese reference works. And Shōzen sometimes needed to identify domestic substitutes for items that might be hard to obtain, or perhaps too expensive.

All in all, Shōzen's writings reveal to us an extensive network of pharmaceutical knowledge and physical products that through clinical testing were incorporated into, and contributed substantial advances in, the Japanese pharmacopoeia.

Chapter 4

LEPROSY, BUDDHIST KARMIC ILLNESS, AND SONG MEDICINE

We do not know how prevalent the disease of *rai* 癩 (in modern times, the term for Hansen's disease or leprosy) was prior to the Kamakura era, and we do not know how common it was even during that era. However, *rai* leprosy and the condition of those who contracted it were significant medical, social, and religious issues during Kajiwara Shōzen's lifetime. The religious and social status of those suffering from it was sufficiently problematic that historians regularly identify *rai* and the response to it as central to understanding issues of discrimination in the medieval era.

In medieval Japan, *rai* was an affliction that contained multiple cultural meanings.[1] The term *rai* was applied to a number of conditions that affected face, torso, and limbs. Symptoms included a variety of sores, hair loss, scaly skin, and loss of fingers and toes. Skeletons from the era reveal that the bones of the arms and legs might also be damaged, but this was not known contemporaneously.[2] While the symptoms of *rai* were unsightly, medical texts, dictionaries, written descriptions, and visual depictions from the era suggest that other skin conditions were just as striking, or repellent, as those of *rai*.[3] For example, a fourteenth-century pharmacist's handbook notes a treatment for horrible sores that have not healed in ten years and that resemble *rai*. Another work refers to untreatable pustulant sores that get worse between the twelfth and twenty-third years, and the person dies.[4]

The label of *rai* evoked strong responses that body condition alone did not. Efforts to control *rai* sufferers ranged from official regulation of communities of *rai* sufferers to active persecution and harassment. They were generally physically marginalized. Contemporary visual sources paint a bleak picture of their lives under shacks and flimsy shelters, begging for food, and ailing. Those who contracted or thought they had contracted *rai* knew that it would permanently affect their social existence.[5] *Rai* was also a powerful metaphor for deserved punishment, and rivals and enemies were excoriated for having it.[6] However, others sought to alleviate the condition of *rai* sufferers. The priest Nichiren (1221–1281) saw *rai* as a positive sign that karmic sins were about to be expiated and preached that sufferers were to be embraced rather than shunned.[7] Medical specialists, even if they felt that *rai* was untreatable, tried to alleviate the suffering by giving at least palliative care.[8] More positively, and, perhaps motivated by their understanding of the stigma attached to *rai* as much as by the medical challenge it posed, physicians also tried to determine whether symptoms were in fact those of *rai.*[9]

The most significant medical efforts to treat *rai* took place at Gokurakuji in Kamakura, and the first medical description of it—the symptoms, the nature of the affliction, and the treatments to be used—is provided by Shōzen. He has one discussion in chapter 34 of the *Ton'ishō* and another in chapter 5 of the *Man'anpō.* However, while these groundbreaking descriptions are obviously important, scholars have tended not to explore Shōzen's writing with much nuance.[10] Nor have they been particularly sensitive to the notion that *rai* contained multiple meanings, that perceptions of it were not monolithic, or that the notion of karmic illness might also be nuanced. By exploring *rai* as a medical issue, I will show not only that the issue of *rai* is more complex than generally represented, but also how ideas of *rai* found in Song medicine led to a substantial reassessment of the disease that invalidated some previous assumptions about it.

SHŌZEN'S DESCRIPTION OF LEPROSY IN THE *TON'ISHŌ*

Shōzen's description of *rai* in chapter 34 of the *Ton'ishō* is the most extensive colloquial description of it that we have for the entire premodern era. Following are two selections from that description. Here is the first selection:

> As to the origins of *rai* ailment, [various theories have been put forward. Namely the notion of] the five *rai* and the eight winds; the conditions that come in one hundred and thirty varieties; that as a result of sinful

karma in previous lives there is just punishment from the gods and the Buddhas; that it is from foods; or that [it is caused by] disharmony of the four elements [earth, water, fire, wind]. In sum, [in order to treat it] one cultivates roots of goodness, performs repentance, and must cultivate the good.

With respect to this Mountain Ailment: There are many varieties and they are not the same, yet they do not differ in that they transform the body. The eyebrows fall off. Here and there and in the same way on the four limbs, the abdomen, the back, and suchlike, there are corrupted ring-wormy spots. The ten digits of the hands and feet drop off. There is no pain from the tingly corrupted spots, which may be colored green, yellow, red, white or black. Bad blood turns into worms [虫], and these consuming worms grow large, eat widely and deeply, and the skin and flesh fall off aggressively. Moxibustion treatment is ineffective. Even inserting needles causes no pain. And [these worms] consume in from the surface of the body down to the depths, then eat their way from the depths of the body and emerge on the surface. On the surface of the skin nothing might appear untoward, as they have eaten into the depths, but if one looks closely the skin is not at all normal. Figuratively speaking, it is like when even if worms have not eaten on the surface of chestnuts, pears, and suchlike, when they eat in the interior depths the color of the surface changes. Further, "passing clouds" that resemble catfish skin stand out on the transformed body and sometimes they become white and starlike. Sometimes the transformed body is blackish and in short order becomes a decayed body. Sometimes [the body] gets thin and is whitish and reddish like sun and moon. The whiteness spreads and is a watery pale [color]. Sometimes small boils appear on the transformed body and gradually become large. Often scabby eczemic sores like gangrenous sores appear. Sometimes [the person feels] cold and heavy. Sometimes [the sores] are no different from places on the body that have been treated by moxibustion. Sometimes they are no different from wounds. Sometimes they suddenly become watery-weepy just like a burn scar. Sometimes they look like the eye of a horse. They rot and fall off, but this makes no difference and they gradually increase. Moreover, the eyeballs of those who contract it turn white, the nose thickens and becomes large, the [finger- and toe-] nails are thin and damaged, and there is no body oil in the hands and feet [i.e., the skin is desiccated]. The face

> becomes lopsided and dried out, or resembles a [rough-barked] rotund pine tree, and the eyebrows drop off.
>
> Even though these many varieties are dissimilar, they are not painful. They manifest differently on the body than the five *rai* and eight winds and such varieties, but just the same they are produced by wind blood worms.[11] Their shapes are described in detail in this and other books and should be looked at there.
>
> First of all, one should determine by looking whether the fennel aspect [茴面] has or has not entered into the body. If it has already entered then treatments cannot be applied, since it is difficult to treat. If it has not yet entered then it can be treated. Knowing this is a secret of physicians. There is a separate oral transmission.[12]

Here is the second selection:

> Oral transmission.
>
> After being contracted, Mountain Ailment becomes pronounced after thirty to fifty days; but it might also take from one year or two years or up to ten or twenty years. Whether it will be mild or severe is not determinable. Mortality consequently will vary. Base people [下賎ノ者] by and large are quickly damaged. In such cases treatment is not applied, since irrespective of poisons or medicines [i.e., it doesn't matter what one does] it draws in the wind, breaks the bones and disorders [the body]. In the case of unbelievers in the realm of poverty, it is a karmic illness [貧道不信者業病也].[13]

From these selections, it is evident that *rai* was a challenging and multifaceted phenomenon. There was no agreement on its etiology—biological, environmental, social, economic, or religious circumstances were all adduced as explanations. How did Shōzen go about treating it?

SHŌZEN'S TREATMENTS FOR LEPROSY IN *TON'ISHŌ*

Treatment for *rai* drew upon the full arsenal of the contemporary medical system, a sure indication that it was an especially challenging problem.

The treatments included medicines, needling and moxibustion, medicinal baths, baths,[14] drawing blood, avoidance of certain foods and activities, and the invocation of spiritual forces. It was assumed that the treatment might continue for an extended period of time. In short, anything and everything was used to treat *rai,* as can be illustrated by looking at some of the elements involved.

Since *rai* symptoms manifested themselves primarily on the surface of the body, most of the treatments accordingly involved external application of ointments, daubs, powders, washes, and medicinal baths. They were designed to treat sores; to combat the pus produced by sores; to provide soothing relief for itchiness, tingling, or inflammation; to cleanse the uncleanness and impurities that had appeared; and even for regrowing hair. Shōzen also prescribes ingested medicines (in which rice wine is a common ingredient) for bodily pain or for alleviating disharmony of the qi.

The materia medica included domestic items and imported items such as the China good Hempwind Oil 大麻風油.[15] We do not know how readily available all items were, but Shōzen notes that some specialty ingredients (such as Red Dragon, musk, or cuckoo) were not that easy to acquire (in which case he recommends that lesser amounts be used in a prescription).[16] Some of the formulas appear to be well-known ones, but many are noted as being oral transmissions or secret knowledge. Treatment protocols and the time periods for treatment regimens are also specified: Individual treatments might last for anywhere up to two hundred days, and patients might undergo treatment for a period of up to three years.

Medicines for treating *rai* appear to have been identified as a result of clinical experience, and chapter 34 starts with five highly recommended ones.[17] The first, Meeting the Transcendent Pill 遇仙丹, is a secret medicine that will bring down red *rai,* a wonder medicine that lowers elevated qi, and one that may be administered to male and female and young and old alike. The second, Miraculous Desirable Chinese-Artichoke Pill 妙好甘露圓, is a secret internal medicine for *rai* and is particularly suitable for treating face-reddening resulting from red *rai* and the reddening of limbs and body. The third, Penetrating Heaven Rebuilding Powder 通天再造散, brings down the various boils and poisonous swellings resulting from *rai.* The fourth, Eight Winds Powder 八風散, harmonizes the qi unbalanced by fevers and disordered blood. The fifth, Nurturing Qi Decoction 養気湯, is a sixteen-ingredient medicine developed specifically for treating Mountain Ailment and that also treats many other illnesses.

Elsewhere, Shōzen notes six internal medicines;[18] five decoction items, the five ingredients for a five-flavor decoction; and medicinal items to be used for medicinal baths (of which there are four different varieties, employing respectively four, six, five, and four ingredients).

Of the first five medicines, Meeting the Transcendent Pill is of note. It contains twelve domestic and imported ingredients: rhubarb, betel husk, Carpesium, Chinese licorice, shield fern, black morning glory, birthwort, betel nut, *torreya* nut, croton, another betel nut, and a palm. It may have been originally a Chinese formula, and was developed especially for treating *rai* (specifically, bringing down Red *rai*). However, it also seems to have been found to be effective in treating a wider range of problems and could be administered to anybody. In the *Man'anpō,* another version of Meeting the Transcendent Pill (containing two fewer ingredients) is praised as a wonder medicine that treats such things as the ten varieties of three worms and nine worms, twenty-one varieties of swellings, 120 varieties of bone-steaming and corpse-transmitted disease, and many others.[19]

Other medicines did not have specific names but were recommended because of the efficacious ingredients from which the medicine was compounded—and perhaps too because the formula was a closely guarded one. One such formula is described thus:

> In the case of cracks that have been impossible to heal, one must combine the ash of human skull and the ash of "black thief" and apply it. Or else one must soften the shell [柄 *kara,* pattern, being a homophone for *kara* 殼, husk, shell] of Red Dragon and apply it. Or else you must soften Red Dragon with earth oil and apply it. As to earth oil, at the place known as Kokkei in Mino Province there is a mountain temple; oil emerges from the ground beneath the feet of the Buddha that is found there. One must soak cotton in this and apply it.[20]

Successful treatment also required that patients look out for their general condition and avoid foods, actions, or behaviors thought to have an adverse impact on the treatment regimen. With respect to foods, which were classified for their efficacious or deleterious effect on the body, Shōzen was drawing upon an established tradition. In fact, chapter 40 of *Ton'ishō* is a listing of the prohibited and permitted foods for forty-three different types of affliction and injury. However, whereas in that chapter Shōzen lists thirteen prohibited and ten recommended food items,[21] his listings in chapter 34 are more extensive. There he lists seventy-seven items that are that prohibited and twenty-two that are permitted,[22] as well as noting five foods that are to be prohibited during one treatment and in the subsequent bathing treatment.[23] He also mentions that one should avoid items that one might lick, pickled items, raw cold items, and hot things.[24] The reason for this disparity between chapters 40 and 34 is not evident, but perhaps chapter 40 presents some standard listings, while the information in chapter 34 reflects working experience.

Various actions and activities were also considered deleterious to the treatment process. Shōzen doesn't explain the rationale for the choices, but perhaps they reflect common perceptions of what might unnecessarily agitate the body and interfere with the treatment regimen and what types of abstinence were required. Yet again, chapter 40 presents briefer information than we find in chapter 34. In chapter 40, Shōzen notes that those being treated for *rai* were to avoid rice wine, anything that drew cold to the body, and sexual relations.[25] In chapter 34, the things to be avoided include the following: When undergoing treatment for cleansing uncleanness and impurities, patients were not to lock eyes with, listen to, or talk to someone with Mountain Ailment, and males undergoing treatment were not to share lodging with a menstruating woman.[26] In addition, a patient snacking on ginger or drinking cloudy rice wine was not to face towards anyone who was afflicted with a Mountain Ailment. Sexual activity was strictly prohibited: If a patient undergoing a one-hundred-day course of treatment should engage in sex even once, then the problem would immediately recur.[27] Shōzen also notes that both men and women were to avoid, for a period of three years, sex, hot foods, and anything else that would make the body disharmonious.[28]

The efficacy of medicines and treatment was also linked to the spiritual mindfulness of the healer and to the assistance of well-known spiritual and healing figures.[29] We might take this as an indication of the difficulty of treating *rai,* for even though at one point in *Ton'ishō* Shōzen suggests that a mantra might be used at any time when administering medicines,[30] the only specific examples of it that I have discovered are found in chapter 34. There we find that part of the treatment for cleansing uncleanness and impurity involves chanting a Healing Buddha mantra, maintaining a mudra, and praying for the assistance of the wondrous

Buddhas.[31] Or, when applying decocted medicines to the patient, the healer is to follow a prescribed regimen, focus his mind, and harness powerful spiritual assistance:

> When one wishes to start treating, on an empty stomach put the boiled medicine into a large earthenware container, put some pill medicine into that, and administer that. After the morning meal the healer is to perform Buddhist abstinence (from eating fish and meat), then usher in the ill person and then with proper dignity chant the Healing Buddha's minor mantra one hundred and twenty times while maintaining a mudra. Then, *Namu Nichigatsu Tōmyō Yakushi Rurikō nyorai* [南無日月燈明薬師瑠璃光如来] "Praise to [the Buddha] Sun and Moon Glow, to the Healing Buddha the Lapis Lazuli Radiance Tathagata" (six repetitions), [then] *Namu Giba Henjaku Yakushi Rurikō nyorai* [南無耆婆扁鵲薬師瑠璃光如来] "Praise to Jīvaka, Bian Que, the Healing Buddha the Lapis Lazuli Radiance Tathagata" (six repetitions). No other words are to be employed. After doing this twelve times, make the ill person naked, then the healer is to start applying [the liquid medicine] all over the body using a hairbrush, starting from the bottom of the left foot if a male and from the bottom of the right foot if a female, and [their] eyes and mouth are to be closed.[32]

SHŌZEN'S ANALYSIS OF LEPROSY IN *TON'ISHŌ*

As a result of his clinical engagement with *rai,* Shōzen eventually was able to diagnose that *rai* was not a monolithic affliction. He discovered that it came in twelve varieties. Reflecting his clinical engagement, he did not refer to them by terms otherwise found in medical texts. Instead, he identified both the overall affliction and each variety with individual vernacular names. *Rai* was referred to as the Mountain Ailment, for reasons that are not explicated. The names for the twelve varieties identify some distinctive symptom of each. Shōzen's descriptions and classifications demonstrate that one of his goals was to bring some coherence to the *rai* phenomenon and to establish a platform for treatment and understanding. In addition, Shōzen was able to demonstrate to his own satisfaction that *rai* was not uniformly a karmic illness, a discovery that would have had obvious implications for social perceptions of the affliction. Here is the adumbration of the twelve varieties:

Even though there are many varieties, the majority can be classified into twelve varieties. As to knowing them:

1. The Mountain Ailment called Worm Sores [虫瘡]: The lower part of the face is blackish reddish, "passing showers" stand out on the body, and worms are eating underneath.
2. The Mountain Ailment called White Mountain [白山]: The entire body becomes white.
3. The Mountain Ailment called Legs Hot Below [脚熱下]: The body, arms, and legs are thin, and the mouth is damaged as with palsy.
4. The Mountain Ailment called Red Star [赤星]: Redness called Red Mountain appears, the body is reddish and sores appear.
5. The Mountain Ailment called Sun Rings [日輪]: The face when facing towards the sun is red, white, black, and yellow.
6. The Mountain Ailment called Moon Rings [月輪]: When facing the moon, the whites of the eyes are like a paper lantern and the mouth is damaged.
7. The Mountain Ailment called Red Grass [赤草]: The face is reddish, it spreads over the muscle, and the [skin of the] face is thick.

   With these seven types of Mountain Ailment, you must compound eighteen types of medicines. Other times the face is reddish and there is elevated qi, and the four limbs are swollen and reddish. The methods of compounding the medicines are written down separately.
8. The Mountain Ailment called River Burning [河焼]: Things break out (on the skin) like fire spreading out, then they rot, and then sores emerge.
9. The Mountain Ailment called Pitted Mountain [愕山]: The arms and legs (hands and feet) are randomly collapsing and being destroyed.
10. The Mountain Ailment called Hot Wind [熱風]: Things like fish scales appear on the face and body, the arms and legs transform, and the body looks a little as it would if one were presenting offerings [i.e., bent over, crouching].
11. The Mountain Ailment called Black Mountain [黒山]: The body transforms, the arms and legs are blackish and thickish, and the cracks do not heal irrespective of whether the person is ambulatory or bedridden.

12. The Mountain Ailment called Gangrenous Mountain [丹山]: Gangrenous sores appear and spread over the body. For these [last] five varieties of Mountain Ailment, you must compound fifteen [types of medicines].[33]

Later in the chapter, in a section recording "oral transmissions," Shōzen elaborates further on the varieties of *rai* and draws attention to four of them that are considered of karmic origin. The names of these four do not correlate with the twelve types noted already, which might suggest that Shōzen was still in the process of understanding *rai* and had not fully organized his knowledge. In any event, here are his comments on karmic *rai:*

> As to *rai* illness, there are twelve varieties, of which four are said to be a karmic illness. They cannot be treated at all. One knows them through close observation. This is extremely secret.
>
> As to the characteristics of White Rai [白癩]: The eyebrows do not fall off, and there is no change in the color of the eyes. The skin of the body is white and is always like fish scales. Things slough off from the body and things like *kose* sores appear below [those sites]. The body is so itchy that at times it seems like the skin will fly off and it is unbearable. There is no medicine [that will treat it], moxibustion can't be applied [does not work], and the agonizing pain increases. The color spreads rapidly and cannot be treated. It is the product of prior karma [先業]. It is the destruction of the heart viscera.
>
> As to the characteristics of Black Rai [黒癩]: The blood resembles ink. It swells up from below the skin, and the blood that emerges is ink-colored. The body is always in agony and hurts from the depths. Body and mind are disordered. If one applies moxibustion, then it splits and collapses from that scar. Even a medicine obtained from a Transcendent has no power to heal it. It is a karmic illness [業病].
>
> As to the characteristics of Dried Skin [干皮]:[34] At the onset the inside of the body is painful, in the way that it would be from the illness of *kakke* [脚気]. Stools do not follow the heart [i.e., there is no control over defecation]. The face is always heavy and swollen. There are blisterlike things on the arms and legs, and when they dry out, yellow fluid weeps

> out and the healed scar stands up like a burn scar and becomes a white spot. The eyebrows quickly fall off. The eyes turn whitish. The entire body is swollen and the person likes to lie down during the day. The skin is swollen and thick, [but] [finger- and toe-] nails do not hurt. Even if one applies moxibustion, [the skin] does not become warm. The person is perpetually fond of lewd activity, just like a horse in the spring. There are no treatments. It is the destruction of the lung viscera.
>
> As to the characteristics of Thin Turnings [薄轉]: Sometimes at the outset the face is swollen. Death is always sudden. The eyebrows gradually become thinner and in particular the color of the eyes changes. Lots of summer hairs like white stars appear in large numbers all over the body, attached fish scales drop off, and sometimes vinegary liquid oozes from beneath them. There are no treatments and it cannot be healed. It is an illness that destroys the liver viscera.[35]

What we most obviously note from Shōzen's analysis of *rai* is that he has determined that it comes in twelve varieties (even though he gives us more than twelve names), that eight of these can be successfully treated, and that four of them cannot be successfully treated because they are karmic illnesses. But what was a karmic illness? And what was the basis for classifying a given illness (or, more broadly, a particular condition of the body) as a product of karma?

THE PROBLEM OF KARMIC ILLNESS

Medieval Japanese were familiar with the notion that the condition of the body (healthy or not healthy, male or female, in wealthy or poor circumstances, of high or low social station, etc.) reflected one's accumulated karma.[36] However, while it was possible to attribute anything and everything—and the mere fact of becoming ill—to the workings of karma,[37] the idea or label of "karmic illness" was more technically applied to a smaller number of conditions and illnesses that were understood to have been contracted because of some specific karmic infraction. Karmic illness was thus a particular subset of illnesses, and that understanding was reflected in Buddhist nosology.

The Buddhist nosology that was most well known in medieval Japan appears to have been that in Zhiyi's (538–597) *Great Calming and*

Contemplation 摩訶止観 (Ja. *Maka shikan,* Ch. *Mohe zhiguan*) of the sixth century.[38] The priest Nichiren,[39] whose writings were widely disseminated, cites it in his 1275 letter, "On Curing Karmic Disease."[40] He notes that "there are six causes of illness: (1) disharmony of the four elements; (2) improper eating or drinking; (3) inappropriate practice of seated meditation; (4) attack by demons; (5) the work of evil spirits; and (6) the effects of karma." He notes, too, that "illness occurs when evil karma is about to be dissipated." And, while karmic illnesses "vary in severity and one cannot make any fixed pronouncements, . . . the gravest illnesses result from the karma created by slandering the Lotus Sutra." Another of Nichiren's letters, "The Treatment of Illness" from 1278, provides additional texture:

> The illnesses of human beings may be divided into two general categories, the first of which is illness of the body. Physical diseases comprise one hundred and one disorders of the earth element, one hundred and one imbalances of the water element, one hundred and one disturbances of the fire element, and one hundred and one disharmonies of the wind element, a total of four hundred and four maladies. These illnesses do not require a Buddha to cure them. Skilled physicians such as [the Indian physicians] Water Holder and Water Carrier, Jivaka, and [the Chinese physician] Bian Que prescribed medicines that never failed to heal physical sickness. The second category is illness of the mind. These illnesses arise from the three poisons and are of eighty-four thousand kinds. They are beyond the healing powers of the two deities and the three ascetics [of Brahmanism] or the six non-Buddhist teachers. Medicines prescribed by [the legendary Chinese physicians] Shennong and Huangdi are even less effective. Illnesses of the mind differ greatly in severity.[41]

Shōzen also was familiar with Zhiyi's nosology. At the very end of chapter 34 of *Ton'ishō,* Shōzen, while not referring by name to the *Great Calming and Contemplation,* notes the following:

> In sum, illnesses are of six varieties. The first is [illness brought about by] the disharmony of the four elements [earth, water, fire, wind]; the second is [illness brought about by] disharmony of diet; the third is [illness brought about by] improperly engaging in seated meditation; the fourth is karmic illness; the fifth is demonic illness; the sixth is illness [brought about by] evil spirits. Of these six types, the two illnesses demonic and

> evil spirit are treated by divine magic, but only if proper reverence to Buddhist teaching is exhibited during the treatment. Seated meditation illness, on the other hand, is treated through seated meditation. Karmic illness is treated by [the person] reflecting and repenting upon their offenses. [Illnesses caused by] disharmony of the four elements and disharmony of the diet are treated by the physician. However, a karmic illness [which is the underlying cause of either of these types] cannot be so treated. As to the four elements, each one of them has one hundred and one varieties, in total thus four hundred and four illnesses, and they arise from the five viscera. The disharmony is that of the four elements earth, water, fire and wind.[42]

Thus, karmic illness was a recognized category of illness, and as we know, some *rai* were in that category. But since not all illnesses were karmic ones, what made an illness a karmic one? Or what made *rai* a karmic illness? Was there a set list, or could new afflictions be added? If afflictions were determined to be karmic, was there a uniform basis for making that determination? In order to get some sense of how karmic illness was understood in Shōzen's time, I will consider some relevant comments contained in two sutras that were widely read in medieval Japan: the *Mahayana Perfection of Wisdom Sutra* 大般涅槃経 *(Mahāparinirvāna Sūtra)* and the *Lotus Sutra* 妙法蓮華経 *(Saddharma Puṇḍarīka Sūtra).*

The *Mahayana Perfection of Wisdom Sutra* adumbrates some conditions that are considered positive karmic rewards: headaches, pain in the eyes, stomach, and back, an untimely death, criticism, slander, lashings, prison or fetters, hunger, and poverty.[43] But these are overshadowed by negative karmic rewards: being reborn as an animal; being born in female form; having evil manners; and having such imperfections of bodily form and sense organs as deafness, blindness, dumbness, retention of urine, or being a hunchback.[44] The *Lotus Sutra* refers to a similar range of conditions. Someone reborn as a jackal will have scabs and sores and only one eye. Someone reborn as a human will have blighted and dull faculties, be puny, vile, bent, crippled, blind, crazed, or deaf. The condition of poverty, want, and all types of decay are also listed as karmic rewards. Karmic consequences can also affect the treatment of the sick. In the case of someone who had slandered the *Lotus Sutra,* even if he became a doctor and had some success, his patients might die from some other malady, and if he suffered from illness, even good medicine would make the condition worse.[45]

The ubiquity of the idea of karmic illness in medieval Japan has, for our purposes, two implications. First, in the case of conditions that may have been congenital (deafness, for example) or that appeared to strike people at random (such as *rai*), the question of why one person and not another may have the affliction would have been an obvious one to ask. Given the state of medical knowledge, it is likely that the notion of karmic illness provided an entirely satisfactory explanation, in much the same way as the idea of hungry ghosts provided a rational explanation for the disappearance of bodily secretions.[46] Our high-ranking warrior and devout Buddhist Hōjō Shigetoki notes that "On the monthly abstinence days, you must not be intimate with any woman. It is said that a child conceived on such a day will be born crippled, or will even become a mortal enemy of its father;[47] or that "Those who have no children must have committed grave offenses in former lives;"[48] or that "should the stepmother commit wrongs, say to yourself, 'She is like that because she is a woman, and that she was born a woman is no doubt a karmic expiation.'"[49]

Second, whether an illness was karmic seems to have weighed on people's minds and raised the issue of the extent to which one should have recourse to medical treatment. After all, if an illness is karmic, what can be done about it? To refer to Nichiren again, while prayer and sincere repentance were recommended for overcoming the karma that might be the origin of the illness, Nichiren always recommended that people continue to use medicines and physicians.[50] One reason for this appears to have been his understanding that karmic illness was a contingent and nuanced phenomenon rather than an inexorable and mechanistic one, as the following suggests:

> I developed diarrhea on the thirtieth day of the twelfth month of last year [1277], and up until the third or fourth day of the sixth month of this year [1278], it grew more frequent by the day and more severe by the month. Just when I was thinking that it must be my immutable karma, you sent me good medicine. Since taking it, my complaint has diminished steadily and is now a mere one-hundredth fraction of its former intensity.[51]

Now, if dedicated Buddhist proselytizers like Nichiren believed that if an illness was successfully treated then it need not be considered a karmic illness, this raises the issue of what physicians might regard as a karmic illness. After all, if they can treat it, it cannot be karmic; and, as Nichiren clearly indicates, the treatment might proceed on the assumption that even if someone thinks an illness is karmic, he may be proven wrong.

As a conceptual matter, Buddhist physicians readily understood karmic illness. However, determining when the label might be applied to a specific condition or affliction (apart from the standard ones listed in sutras) was not a simple matter. It appears that while afflictions were labeled as karmic, there were no common guidelines for determining what would qualify (or, alternately, not qualify) something as a karmic illness, so physicians used their own judgment and discretion. Thus not only was the treatment of karmic illness uncertain, so too was the use of the concept. The following four elements were in play when physicians engaged karmic illness.

First (and as we already know from the case of *rai*), medieval physicians were certain that karmic illnesses existed. They classified a number of ailments as karmic (or not) and were aware that medicine might not be efficacious because the affliction was a karmic illness. For example, the author of the fourteenth-century *Gotai miwakeshū* 五体身分集 (Collection on the Five Portions of the Body) notes that a type of White-hot Wind is *not* a karmic illness; another section notes that the affliction Water Sea, where the belly swells, the skin glistens, and the person dies within five years, is an immutable karmic illness 常業ノ病.[52] In the *Ton'ishō,* Shōzen notes that a newly arrived work lists a medicine that is successful in treating infant and child depression (and is particularly efficacious if the woman breastfeeding the infant also drinks it) and that except in those cases where the condition is the result of an immutable karmic illness, it is effective in ninety-nine out of a hundred people.[53]

Second, since physicians did not have a shared basis for making their assessment of something as a karmic illness, they might make different diagnoses for the same afflictions. One clear example of this emerges from a comparison of two treatises on corpse-transmitted disease written by Buddhist priests in the early fourteenth century. The first was compiled by Kōshū in 1318.[54] The second, the *Denshibyō nijūgo hō* 伝屍病二十五方 (Twenty-Five Methods for Treating Corpse-Transmitted Diseases), was compiled by Gahō in 1334.[55] Kōshū makes no note of the source of his information, but Gahō says that he had received his information from a Chinese physician. The works are virtually identical. Both focus on moxibustion as the preferred treatment; both designate twenty-five varieties (the first item is a general description of the overall category) of corpse-transmitted diseases; allowing for obvious transcription errors, the names of the twenty-five varieties are almost all the same; and they agree that the afflictions are fatal if untreated, some fatal even if treated, and that the period between contraction and death differs among the varieties.

The two works differ primarily in their assessment of whether any of the varieties comprised a karmic illness. Kōshū notes that variety number three is a karmic illness, and that variety eleven is a karmic illness of the qi 気業. By contrast, Gahō notes that of the twenty-five, numbers three, eight, thirteen, and twenty-five are karmic in nature, and that number eleven is not karmic in nature. Given that the two works exhibit little disagreement over the naming, the order in which they are listed, the descriptions, and the treatments, it is difficult to know how or why the two authors had such different understanding over which might be classified as karmic illnesses. They agree on only one, there is some overlap on another, and one author designates three illnesses that had not been so designated by the other. Neither tells us what about any of them made them karmic illnesses. And, even though we might speculate that a designation of karmic illness might have been based on the affliction not being amenable to treatment, this does not explain why other varieties that were likewise deemed untreatable would not have been given the karmic designation. We are thus left with the simple fact that two authors describing the same afflictions disagree on designations of karmic illness. This suggests that the category of karmic illness was one of convenience rather than one of uniform explanatory efficacy.

Third, the idea of karmic illness was used in order to interpret, or make meaningful, characterizations found in Chinese medical works. An example here is Shōzen's understanding of the variety of colic known as genital colic—primarily an affliction of males, with symptoms such as painful swellings in the abdomen, small intestine, bladder, or scrotum and testicles. It came in four different varieties: intestinal colic, colic of the qi, water colic, and egg colic.[56] In trying to understand genital colic, Shōzen drew on the *Yanshi jisheng fang* (Mr. Yan's Formulas for Benefiting Life) of 1253, the *Taiping Shenghui fang* of 992, and the *Sanyin fang* of 1174. The *Sanyin fang* concluded that when infants suffer from egg colic, it must be regarded as a lodged disease 宿疾.[57] However, while essentially borrowing the phrasing of the *Sanyin fang* for his description, Shōzen tried to make sense of lodged disease by interpreting it in a Buddhist framework and understanding it to mean lodged or residual karma 宿業. He notes in the *Ton'ishō* that "Further, in the case of infants it is something with which they are born (innate disposition), and as they get older it is lodged colic and is there because of residual karma. Of these four types of genital colic, egg colic and intestinal colic are difficult to treat, while colic of the qi and water colic are easy to treat."[58] And in the *Man'anpō* two decades later, he notes that "Further, where we have an infant and after birth it becomes like this, then it is a lodged illness, i.e., it is an illness of residual karma."[59]

Fourth, we encounter instances where the idea of karmic illness is not applied, even when it may have been possible to do so, because another explanation was more encompassing. An example here is Shōzen's assessment of corpse-transmitted disease. In the *Ton'ishō,* Shōzen notes such things as there are at least six variant terms for corpse-transmitted disease; different sources note it as having twenty-two, thirty-six, or even ninety-nine varieties; it is usually transmitted from corpses; a person can get it from relatives; there are a variety of causes from which it arises; there are a variety of symptoms; and that throwing the body into a river will wash the transmission away.[60] Significantly, Shōzen has absolutely no reference to karma or karmic illness.

The *Man'anpō* commentary on corpse-transmitted disease (specifically on the variety known as depletion) draws on chapter 4 of the early Yuan work Sun Rencun's *Rencun Sunshi zhibing huofa mifang* 仁存孫氏治病活法秘方 (Rencun Mr. Sun's Secret Formulas for Treating Disease and Techniques for the Living).[61] There we find that corpse-transmitted diseases are caused by worms that inhabit the viscera and that upon the death of the host, the worms move to new hosts (such as family members) that had been in proximity to the victim. Acccording to the text, the worms came in several colors, affected different viscera, and were manifested in different symptoms. There were a total of nine worms, of which three were generally known, being intestinal worms, parasites, and stomach worms. The other six were new types of worms. Whereas stomach worms needed no explanation as to location and shape, the new ones are described in the text, and the description is accompanied by an illustration.[62]

However, while the notion of worms provided an explanation of how the affliction operated as a physical phenomenon, the question of why somebody may have become afflicted still remained. Sun Rencun surmised that it might be due to such things as the accumulation of karma from ancestors who had killed, destiny having accumulated into this world, having been steeped in evil habits that have yet to be expunged and for which later people have not been forgiven, or not taking care of ancestral graves or properly performing rites.[63] Now, while Sun Rencun does not use the term "karmic illness," it might have been possible for Shōzen to remark that corpse-transmitted disease was a karmic illness. After all, medieval Japanese saw the Chinese notion of destiny as equivalent to the Buddhist concept of karma,[64] and Shōzen was aware, for example, that whether an infant might live or what its lifespan might be was determined at birth.[65] However, even though (as we know) other contemporary physicians had suggested that at least some corpse-transmitted diseases were karmic illnesses, Shōzen makes no reference to this at all. It is entirely likely then that Shōzen had concluded that Sun Rencun's notion of worms was a medically more nuanced explanation than a default recourse to karma.

In sum, karmic illness was an accepted category. Yet it is evident that for physicians and thus as a medical matter, karmic illness was a useful but malleable category. Afflictions could be assessed as karmic, but there was no uniform standard for such determinations. Physicians might disagree over the status of the same afflictions. Physicians might also, on the basis of new explanations, come to feel that it did not make much sense to regard something as a karmic illness. Given this variation, then, we may not be surprised to find a physician going one step further and concluding that the idea of karmic illness might no longer provide a satisfactory explanation for an affliction.

OBSERVATIONS ON LEPROSY IN THE *MAN'ANPŌ*

I now turn to Shōzen's views on *rai* made in the *Man'anpō* a quarter of a century after he made his comments in the *Ton'ishō.* In the *Man'anpō, rai* is taken up in chapter 5, titled "Section Dealing with the Various Winds Related to Horrible Rai" (which the index notes is colloquially referred to as "Mountain Ailment").[66] *Rai,* obviously, is thus categorized as one of the afflictions caused by winds. While it is commonly remarked that the chapter devoted to *rai* in the *Ton'ishō* is given special status in that it is not placed in the traditional category of wind-caused ailments, insofar as chapter 5 of the *Man'anpō* is obviously devoted primarily to *rai* this surely indicates that even within the winds category, *rai* was considered as an entity in itself. More to the point, it suggests that Shōzen had come to the conclusion that *rai* indeed belonged in the winds category, whereas in the *Ton'ishō* the etiology was less clear.

There are some obvious differences between Shōzen's presentation of *rai* in *Ton'ishō* and *Man'anpō.* The first of these relates to the sources that he consulted. In the *Ton'ishō,* Shōzen does not indicate by name any written sources. From the phrasing in the *Ton'ishō,* however, we can identify at least three (assuming that Shōzen saw them directly and did not cite from something else). As noted earlier, he cites the Buddhist treatise *Great Calming and Contemplation.* The second source is Sun Simiao's *Beiji qianjin yaofang* (Priceless and Essential Formulas for Emergencies), from which Shōzen selects some phrasing in the section on "Horrible Afflictions Great Winds" 悪疾大風 that appears in the chapter "Fistulas and Oozing."[67] The third source is the chapter on wind disorders in Wang Huaiyin's 王懐隠 *Taiping Shenghui fang* (Formulas of Great Peace and Sagely Benevolence);[68] while Shōzen borrows phrasing, it is clear that he selected them rather than simply copying out larger passages. Otherwise, it is clear that the discussions and descriptions in the *Ton'ishō* are based on direct clinical experience.

By contrast, in the *Man'anpō* the descriptions of *rai,* classification of types of *rai,* and medicines used are drawn almost exclusively from two Chinese texts, the *Shengji zonglu* and the *Sanyin fang.* And, while Shōzen puzzlingly does not even mention the *Shengji zonglu* by name, the structure of the chapter essentially replicates chapter 18 of that work (it does omit a section on "white patch," or *vitaligo*)[69] and adds to that at the end some material from the *Sanyin fang.* Since the *Shengji zonglu* came to Shōzen's attention only subsequent to the completion of the *Ton'ishō,* this suggests that Shōzen—informed of course by his clinical experience in treating *rai*—had determined that the information in the *Shengji zonglu* provided a better understanding of *rai* than what he had provided in the *Ton'ishō.* Here I will comment on the overall structure, on formulas and medicines, and on explanations for *rai* that appear in the *Man'anpō.*

Chapter 5 of *Man'anpō* has nine sections (with the material from the *Sanyin fang* constituting in effect an unnumbered addendum). Three sections deal with non-*rai* skin afflictions. Six are on the *rai* topics of Horrible Wind (noted as being *rai* illness, which the *Man'anpō* index notes is colloquially referred to as *kataki*), the falling off of eyebrows and hair due to Great Wind (Shōzen notes that this is the overall name for *rai,* and that it is also referred to as Hempwind), worms produced by Great Wind (the index notes that the five types of worms enter the five viscera and cause the illness), Great Wind *rai* illness, Crow (black) *rai,* and White *rai.* The information, as noted, is drawn verbatim from the *Shengji zonglu,* Shōzen has no comments of his own, and none of the material that is found in the *Ton'ishō* is included here. The only overlap with named types of *rai* that appear in the *Ton'ishō* is with Black *rai* and White *rai*, which in *Ton'ishō* are considered karmic varieties of *rai*.

The material on medicines in chapter 5 is also presented quite differently than it is in the *Ton'ishō*. There are no references to oral traditions or secret transmissions, there is no reference to secret or unwritten compounding instructions, there are no references to mantras or to the need to call for the assistance of other healing forces or figures when administering or applying medicine, and there is no mention of things to be avoided when taking medicine or when undergoing treatment. Instead, the only medicines that are mentioned have specific names, and they are drawn only from the *Shengji zonglu*, the *Sanyin fang*, and the *Hejiju fang*.

It is also clear that the medicines included are ones that he had used clinically. In a number of instances, Shōzen adjusted the original formula. For example, whereas the *Shengji zonglu* notes there are to be fifteen to twenty pills in a dose of Chinese Cornbind Pill 何首烏丸, Shōzen notes that it is to be twenty to thirty, and if that doesn't work then the dose should be increased to fifty to sixty pills.[70] In another instance, he adds some medicines to a list of those that are to be used in treating a problem.[71] For another formula, he increases the frequency with which a dose is to be taken; for example, instead of two doses during the day, he suggests two or three doses during the day.[72] And in another case, not only does Shōzen increase the amount of the daily dose, he expands the period of imbibing salty rice wine from one hundred days to two to three years, and with respect to the supplemental use of moxa six months after the beginning of treatment, he increases the number of moxa cones to be used per application from fourteen (two sevens) to thirty to fifty.[73] Whereas we do not know how many medicines Shōzen may have tried and not included in the *Ton'ishō*, in the *Man'anpō* we have a clearer sense. In addition to including two medicines from the *Hejiju fang*,[74] Shōzen included 28 of the 133 medicines listed in the *rai* section of the *Shengji zonglu* and three of the twelve medicines listed in the equivalent section of the *Sanyin fang*. Given Shōzen's intense interest in finding effective medicine for treating *rai* and knowing his penchant for clinically testing medicines, we may assume at the very minimum that he had come to the conclusion that of all the possible medicines and treatments with which he was familiar, thirty-three were the most efficacious, and that those formulas (of which

84 percent were from the *Shengji zonglu*) were to be found in only three Chinese medical works.

With respect to the causes of *rai,* whereas in the *Toni'shō* Shōzen presents a range of theories, in the *Man'anpō* he presents a clear theory. That theory is that bad winds are of five types that impact all of the qi. Those winds have five colors (green, white, red, black, and yellow), and when these poisons enter into the five viscera they produce worms, which are of five types. Those worms in turn dig into the marrow and the five viscera, and they also eat the qi and blood and inflict damage. That damage is manifested in different symptoms, such as eyebrows falling off, nose collapsing, disordered speech, ringing in the ears, itchiness and sores on the skin, sweating, transformation of the face, drying out of the skin, and numerous different types of damage to the skin.[75]

In accepting the notion of *rai* being caused by winds and the worms they produce, Shōzen unmistakably moved away from the idea that karma was somehow involved in *rai.* In the *Ton'ishō,* Shōzen pointed out that there were twelve types of *rai,* only four of which were karmic, so already he was predisposed to the idea that karma did not explain all *rai.* In the *Man'anpō,* Shōzen moves a step further, adopting the position that karma does not explain any *rai.* The evidence for this is Shōzen's inclusion of a passage from the *Sanyin fang* dealing with White *rai* (which in the *Ton'ishō* was one of the *rai* considered to be a karmic illness).[76] The *Sanyin fang* passage touches on the possibility of White *rai* being caused by karma resulting from inhumanity and the most unimaginable lewdness, but then it rejects that position, asking how it is possible for something that is transmitted by qi and blood to be the product of residual karmic bonds. Presumably, if Shōzen felt that this dismissal of a karmic explanation for *rai* was mistaken, then he would have remarked on it. Yet he did not.

SOME CONCLUDING COMMENTS

Rai was a medically challenging affliction, and it appears to have been perceived as a karmic illness. However, while *rai* was not the only affliction that was determined as being karmic in nature, it appears to have been the only one to have elicited an identifiable range of negative perceptions that resulted in discriminatory social behavior towards its sufferers. Yet the clinical activities of Shōzen, and no doubt innumerable others, indicate that another response was to provide care and medical treatment in an effort to cure the problem or at the minimum to alleviate the symptoms. Clearly, discriminatory responses were not the only ones, which calls into question monolithic characterizations of the affliction in the medieval era.

The idea of karmic illness, while regarded as a valid interpretative category, was not, however, straightforward. Positively, the notion could provide a convincing explanation for afflictions whose etiologies were unclear, where the affliction was contracted apparently randomly and with no necessarily evident relationship to a person's social or environmental circumstances (that is, it was unclear why *this* person rather than *that* person contracted it), it was difficult to treat, and where there was little sign of the symptoms being ameliorated or arrested. Problematically, while examples of karmic afflictions were listed in Buddhist texts, there was otherwise no prior list among physicians of what afflictions might fall under the rubric of karmic illness. As the example of corpse-transmitted diseases makes abundantly clear, there was no general agreement on what symptoms would justify labeling something as karmic or not. Even more revealing, as we saw anecdotally in the case of Nichiren and as a result of clinical experience in the case of Kajiwara Shōzen, successful treatment of symptoms was sufficient grounds for people to reject a prior determination that an affliction might have a karmic basis. For Shōzen—well aware of the negative social connotations engendered by *rai* and motivated by the fundamental Buddhist injunction to heal—clinical engagement of *rai* implicitly held out the possibility that it might prove treatable. That is, *rai* need not be accepted as simply karmic.

In short, towards the end of his life and after many decades of clinical exposure to *rai,* Shōzen the Buddhist physician appears to have made a significant intellectual leap. In the case of one of the most vexing medical and social problems of his day, he came to the conclusion that understandings rooted in Buddhist notions of karma and karmic illness were less useful than understandings deriving from interpretations based on more recent advances in Chinese medicine.

Chapter 5

WARFARE, WOUND MEDICINE, AND SONG MEDICAL KNOWLEDGE

The preceding chapters have looked at the engagement of Song medical knowledge in a time of peace. The environment was conducive to acquiring books, to gauging the efficacy of medicines, and to spending extended periods of time reflecting upon medicine, and it facilitated ready access to a wide range of materia medica. In 1333, however, four years before Kajiwara Shōzen's death, that environment changed radically.

While the details need not detain us here, an unprecedented explosion of violence resulted, for the first time in Japanese history, in the obliteration of an entire institution of government. The Kamakura *bakufu* was destroyed, the governing Hōjō warrior dynasty was virtually eliminated as over a thousand males were killed in battle or in spectacular scenes of self-immolation, and much of the city of Kamakura was reduced to ashes. A society that had relied upon the force of authority became one that relied upon the authority of force, and warfare became one of the distinguishing characteristics of Japanese society for nearly three centuries thereafter.[1]

For our purposes, the most important by-product of the fighting in the fourteenth century was that, even though Japan's warrior class had been in existence for some centuries, battle wounds were for the first time incurred with sufficient frequency and in sufficiently large numbers to prompt the emergence of wound medicine as a specialty. The first works on wound medicine, the anonymous *Kinsō ryōjishō* 金瘡療治抄 (On Healing Incised Wounds) of 1356 or 1357,[2] and Tominikōji Norizane's

富小路範實 *Kihō* 鬼法 (Demon Formulas) of 1391,[3] were thus written in specific historical circumstances, and changes in the nature of warfare were directly linked to developments in Japanese medicine. These circumstances also provide us with an opportunity to see another range of factors that shaped the appropriation of Song medicine in the medieval era. As will be seen, while knowledge about the treatment of wounds gained from printed books was minimal, the conceptual understanding of wound medicine was provided by a Song author, and materia medica associated with Song medicine was an integral part of wound treatment.

THE NEW WARFARE ENVIRONMENT FROM THE 1330S

From 790 there was no standing Japanese army, but there were also no domestic or foreign threats to guard against. There was thus no formal infrastructure for training, instruction in strategy, military engineering, or combat medical services. Weapons and armor were produced by a limited number of craft specialists. Internal security was provided by a self-equipped provincial warrior elite that served mainly as local officials within a framework of civil administration.[4] The rare armed conflict that occurred was limited geographically and primarily took the form of skirmishes and ad hoc campaigns.[5] While fighting was prosecuted with verve and was unconstrained by notions of chivalry, it was rarely pursued to bloody conclusion.[6] Even the nationwide fighting of the 1180s that ushered in the Kamakura *bakufu* was less a concerted mobilization than a series of campaigns punctuated by local score-settling, though it did end with a destructive pacification expedition against a regional power center in 1189 (after which the army was disbanded).[7] The fighting against the Mongols in 1274 and 1281, while intense, was of limited duration.[8] Finally, participation in conflict was essentially limited to members of the warrior class.

The fighting in 1332 and 1333 that led to the destruction of the Kamakura *bakufu* in mid-1333 ushered in an epochal change in the nature of military conflict in Japan: Battles and campaigns were replaced by the larger phenomenon of warfare.[9] Four elements in particular illustrate the way in which the nature of fighting changed. First, conflict was pursued with a greater intensity than previously. We note periods of fighting when a larger proportion of wounds were inflicted by close-in weapons such as swords, in contrast to the standoff weapon of the bow and arrow that had previously dominated the battlefield. The practice of suicide in the face of defeat became common. Extended sieges of fixed fortifications, a new development, usually resulted not in surrender or the abandoning of the siege but in starvation, cannibalism, fighting to the last, and execution of survivors.[10] Second, campaigning occurred in all seasons and in all weather conditions. Cold-weather fighting required treatment for people being pulled from freezing rivers ("autumn frost ripped their flesh, the dawn ice stuck to their skin")[11] and exposed troops to frostbite and hypothermia, and troops who found themselves and their horses stuck in the snow or unable to string their bows properly because of frozen fingers found themselves easy targets for better-equipped opponents.[12] Third, reflecting a new battle mentality where the goal was not simply victory but to inflict as much bodily harm as possible, almost anything that could be used as a weapon was employed. The weapons normally associated with the samurai—the sword and bow and arrow—were augmented by spears (which made their first recorded appearance in 1334), iron clubs, rocks, boiling water, logs, fire, and burning oil.[13] In part, this new range of weapons reflects the fact that the demand for the traditional weapons, produced by artisans in small quantities, outstripped the supply of them. It also reflects the fact that fighting was no longer restricted to members of the warrior class but now included virtually all segments of society: Commoners might be recruited into armies or forced to take up weapons to defend themselves against depredation and, in the worst cases, random head-hunting. Fourth and finally, there was the emergence of a new calculus of reward for service, by which the evidence of actual wounds was privileged over mere presence on the battlefield.[14] This did not mean that warriors intentionally went into battle in order to become injured, but it did mean that warriors were given added incentive to actively participate in fighting, which of course increased the likelihood of being wounded.

Warriors have left us considerable information on the injuries they received in the form of battle service reports.[15] These documents range in coverage from a note that a person was wounded[16] to a recounting of injuries suffered over a week or so of fighting by a large number of people serving in one detachment[17] to lists of wounds incurred by family members over the course of a year.[18] They do not always describe the state of a wound itself, and we do not have much information on wounds for which treatment may have been received but which proved fatal, but they do provide detail that is not available for any other area of contemporary medicine.[19]

From battle service reports we learn such things as the names of the injured individuals, the number of injuries received by a person, the location on the body of the injury, how many in a group may have suffered injury, and the date and the geographical location where the injury was suffered, and the documents also provide scholars with rich material to interpret the relationship between injuries received and the weapons and armor employed.[20] We can deduce from the documents that most survivable wounds were to the bodily extremities; that most were liable to have been caused by blades and arrows; and that, while we have instances where people suffered multiple wounds,[21] most combatants were likely to be wounded only once in any encounter. We have few references to people suffering serial wounds,[22] but since warriors were exposed to battle over an extended period of time, there was a concomitant high likelihood of being wounded at some point. Warriors may not have been able to depend upon a period of recuperation before having to fight again and would sometimes continue fighting while wounded.[23] The number of casualties that might result from an encounter varied. Some battles produced large numbers; on other occasions, the wounded were a small percentage of those who fought.[24]

All in all, the expectation of warriors was that at some point they would be wounded and would need treatment. The shift from peacetime to wartime and the sudden growth in the need for emergency trauma treatment would pose a challenge at any time. But in fourteenth-century Japan, there was an additional challenge: Namely, until this time wound medicine was not an area of particular expertise. Let us look at how that expertise developed and at the factors influencing the contributions of Song medical knowledge.

WOUND MEDICINE BEFORE THE 1330S

Prior to the 1330s, battle casualties seem to have been far fewer than the claims that embellish literary sources.[25] But visual depictions of battle injury—arrow wounds to the head, the lower leg, in or near the eye, or through the neck from front to back, and images of a warrior whose leg had been sliced off below the knee or of a severed forearm lying on the ground—leave no doubt that wounds would need to be treated.[26] However, battlefield medical care seems to have been fairly rudimentary. Written sources refer to simply attending to the wounded and only specifically mention the use of moxibustion.[27] Visual sources illustrate such things as an arrow being extracted from the face using something like a large set of tweezers, the tending of shoulder and chest wounds, or a warrior bandaging the head wound of another.[28] We also have a few scattered references to the effects of injury on warriors, such as those that made it difficult or impossible to wield a sword normally,[29] being unable to see properly,[30] becoming lame in one leg as a result of an arrow wound,[31] or being left with a hoarse voice as a result of an arrow wound to the windpipe.[32]

We also have references to trauma injuries in peacetime. For example, a disturbance at an archery competition in Kamakura resulted in three people being wounded, one person being killed, two hit by practice arrows, and one person trampled to death by a horse.[33] Acts of violence also produced injuries that needed treatment, such as those inflicted in one notorious case by a warrior who, among other forms of harassment, tied women behind horses and dragged them around a village and cut off the ears and sliced off the noses of women and children.[34] A round of rural violence in 1259 left one female victim barely alive after being cut in numerous places; we learn that she had to spend at least twenty days prostrate and abed, received moxibustion treatment, and although she "revived," there was so little hope for her recovery that she entered holy orders.[35] One might also safely assume that the normal rhythms of an agricultural society would have produced injuries that required treatment.

Despite the obvious need to treat injury, however, there is very little evidence that trauma medicine was regarded as a specialty area, and there are very few references to people who may have had any skills in that area. In an example from the Jōkyū war of 1221, a monk provided treatment to a warrior wounded by an arrow: Grass leaves were rubbed together, the warrior swallowed them, blood drained from his stomach, his body was lightened, and he felt better. However, the efficacy of the treatment had less to do with medical techniques than it did with the healing powers of a statue of the Healing Bodhisattva Yakushi Kannon to whom the warrior had made pilgrimage in the past.[36]

Two other examples suggest that some treatment for wounds could involve controversial techniques and medicines. In a case dated to 972–974, a doctor informs a warrior that, since his sore is much the same as a wound, he should use the medicine known as Dried Infant (which is a powder medicine derived from an aborted or miscarried fetus), and that it should be that of a male rather than female infant.[37] A second example comes from 1198, and in this case also the healer prescribes Dried Infant, much to the disgust of a shrine priest who considered it the same as eating a dead person. This case is of additional interest because it provides our first reference to someone who claims to be a specialist in treating blade injuries 疵医師.[38] No doubt there were other healers who claimed expertise in treating ailments and had skills that might be applied to dealing with wounds—such as the Chinese tooth puller in Nara, or the spectacularly unsuccessful self-proclaimed specialist in eye problems who appears in the illustrated *Yamai no sōshi* 病の草紙 (Scroll of Afflictions).[39] While we have no way of knowing the source of their training or their knowledge, we are probably on safe ground in assuming that such individuals were either self-taught or had received oral instruction and had but slight acquaintance with written texts.

Turning to physicians associated with more learned traditions of healing, we also find little evidence of special interest in wound medicine. Physicians employed at the imperial court tended to the needs of a sedentary aristocracy whose activities were rarely of the type that might result in traumatic injuries. Court physicians focused on such matters as reproduction and childbirth, enteric problems, food poisoning, colds, and diabetes (though not understood as such at the time).[40] Physicians employed by the Kamakura *bakufu* were recruited from among the ranks of these court physicians.[41] Members of the Tanba family may have had some knowledge of external injury, since chapter 18 of the *Ishinpō* (to which they presumably had access) deals with wounds, burns, incised wounds, arrow wounds, falling from a horse, dog bites, and horse bites.[42] However, it seems that the Kamakura *bakufu,* though a warrior government, saw little need for skills in the treatment of wounds, and the physicians served the domestic needs of the shogunal household.

This apparent lack of clinical interest in or experience with trauma injury is also attested in the *Ton'ishō.* Even though it is directed to physicians who did not normally have access to medical writings, contains much information from oral sources, and was well regarded by important warriors in Kamakura, as far as I can tell it has only two references to treating wounds. The first reference is in chapter 24, which deals with various types of boils, carbuncles, and sores. When noting the formula Divine Efficacy Chinese-Angelica Ointment 神効當皈膏, Shōzen comments that it was good for regrowing flesh on the scars of sores or wounds *(mono no kasa kizu no ato).*[43] The second example appears in chapter 40, which lists permitted and prohibited foods for patients being treated for any of forty-three separate types of afflictions. One section of that chapter is devoted to enumerating the foods that are permitted or not for those undergoing treatment for incised injury, which shows that Shōzen was aware that wounds belonged in their own category of treatment.[44] However, while virtually all of the other forty-two afflictions that are listed in chapter 40 are elsewhere in the *Ton'ishō* allocated separate chapters or at least an individual section of a chapter, there is nowhere a chapter or section separately devoted to the treatment of wounds. As will be noted, however, the *Ton'ishō* does nevertheless contain a great deal of information and recommendations for the treatment of various other conditions that might be extended to the treatment of wounds.

In the *Man'anpō,* in contrast, Shōzen does devote a separate chapter to the treatment of trauma injury: chapter 24. The title of the chapter, "Incised Injuries" 金瘡, replicates the title of a chapter in the *Shengji zonglu.* While some of the works that Shōzen used when compiling the *Man'anpō* (such as *Hejiju fang, Puji benshi fang,* or *Shizhai baiyi xuanfang*) have chapters or sections of chapters devoted to incised injury, Shōzen doesn't draw on them.[45] This would seem to suggest that his decision to include this chapter was prompted by the fact that *Shengji zonglu* had a separate chapter devoted to the subject. One should not underestimate the importance of identifying incised injuries as an area of treatment requiring its own knowledge, but it does not appear that in including it Shōzen was responding to any pressing need. For one thing, the chapter is among the shortest in the *Man'anpō.* For another, whereas throughout both the *Ton'ishō* and the *Man'anpō* he has comments that suggest he was directly familiar with the medical issue involved and was well acquainted with the formulas, in this chapter I can find only one such suggestion. And that comment—that he had found a certain medication effective at stopping the pain from hot water burns—does not deal with incised injury but with an external trauma that might be encountered in the course of daily life.[46] (Parenthetically, the only other comment on wounds that I have encountered in *Man'anpō* is likewise partly related to daily life: He notes in chapter 62 that Japanese pears are not to be eaten by those who have suffered wounds or by expectant women).[47]

The structure and composition of chapter 24 also suggest that Shōzen did not have much direct familiarity with injuries caused by weapons. The chapter is divided into eleven sections that cover the topics of treatments for the following: when bleeding does not stop; incised injury to flesh and bone; feverishness caused by incised injury; palsy resulting from incised injury; viscera emerging as a result of incised injury; injury caused by poison arrows (which Shōzen notes are called *busuya* in Japan);[48] injury caused by arrow blades in the flesh; injuries from bamboo or wood where the slivers won't come out; incised injury where the intestines are protruding; injuries resulting from falls from great heights, horses, and carriages; and burns caused by hot water and fire. The first eight of the eleven sections draw exclusively from the two relatively brief chapters (139 and 140) in the *Shengji zonglu* that cover incised injury and arrow injury. Shōzen has done little more than engage in some editorial selection and rearrangement. The remaining three sections, on the other hand, draw their information from a range of works. Section 9 draws mainly on the the *Keyong fang* (treating incised injuries) but also references the *Shengji fang* (incised wounds where intestines have been cut). In section 10 he draws on *Hejiju fang* (falls from horses), the *Jianyi fang* (falls from a high place), and the *Yuyaoyuan fang*.[49] Section 11, on hot water and fire injuries, draws on the *[Huoren] Shizheng fang houji*.

To sum all of this up then, as late as 1327, when the *Man'anpō* was completed, Shōzen did not see any pressing clinical reason to focus on weapon injuries. The strong implication is that he did not expect that his readers would need to have any detailed knowledge of treatment for wound and trauma injury. More broadly, just before the outbreak of warfare in the 1330s, wound medicine was not identified as an area requiring particular attention. One cannot identify any demand for people with specialized knowledge of wound injury, there are only sporadic references to people who claimed some special skill in that area, and as far as I can tell there were no manuals or compilations that might handily encapsulate any available knowledge.

SOURCES OF KNOWLEDGE FOR WOUND MEDICINE

In 1333, physicians lacked the knowledge, training, and facilities to deal with the range and number of battle injuries that accompanied the descent into a civil war that was to last for over half a century. But they responded to the need, no doubt through trial and error, and built up a fund of relevant knowledge. Wound medicine became a new area of medical expertise, and by the 1390s at the latest, wound physicians had become integral members of warrior households and were on call to treat the highest ranking members of society.[50] The knowledge of injuries and treatments that lay behind that expertise is written down in two specialist works—the *Kinsō ryōjishō* of 1356 or 1357 and the *Kihō* of 1391—and their tables of contents convey the gist of that knowledge. Following is the table of contents from the *Kinsō ryōjishō:*

1. Knowing whether the wound is fatal
2. The ten good and the ten bad signs
3. Stopping the blood from a wound
4. Knowing the pain of a wound
5. Stopping blood awryness
6. Putting back in viscera that have come out
7. Making blood seep from a wound that is not seeping
8. Expelling blood that has lodged in the body
9. Opening the mouth of a wound
10. Stopping delirium as a result of the wound
11. Extracting an arrowhead that has become lodged
12. Mending shins, forearms, and trunks that have been severely cut
13. Mending muscle/sinew that has been cut
14. A separate oral transmission for mending necks that have been cut
15. Where wounds are drawing away life
16. Fixing where [an arrowhead?] is lodged in the mouth of an injury
17. So that wounds are not swollen and not suppurating
18. A wound where the surface is healed but the underneath is not healed
19. Treating palsy [中風] and *kakke* [脚気] resulting from the injury
20. Healing wounds that have become suppurative
21. Treating for when wounds are leading towards *kakke*
22. Treating for arrow piercing where the mouth of the injury is narrow and the base [of the injury] is deep
23. Where the mouth of the wound is rolled inwards and [the person] will die
24. How to know the depth or shallowness of a wound
25. Special wounds that suddenly heal in a night
26. Wounds where the flesh suddenly heals and grows back
27. Healing wounds that have not healed over a long period
28. Flaring up of old wounds as a result of improper [悪] activities
29. Insects [maggots, worms] appearing in a wound

30. Being struck with a poisoned arrow
31. Mending genitals that have been cut
32. Washing wounds
33. Healing wounds without [leaving] scars
34. Making indented scars flat
35. Regrowing [flesh] where flesh has been lost
36. Treating where the healed mouth of a wound has become raised
37. Removing the sweet flesh [甘肉] on a wound
38. Making attractive a wound [scar] on the head
39. Brains protruding from a wound to the head
40. When legs are unsteady as the result of a head wound
41. When someone is bent up due to the wounds
42. Blood coming from the throat as a result of a wound
43. Treating for when there are sudden changes in the eyes [due to] pain within the body [from] the injury
44. Wound medicine
45. [Foods] poisonous and medicinal for wounds
46. Treating wounds with moxibustion
47. Having been wounded, where death is certain
48. Wounds to the nails
49. Purgative medicines [to relieve constipation as a result of a wound]
50. Treating with *candock*
51. Making seep from an arrow wound blood that is not seeping
52. Stopping life [息] from coming out of a wound
53. Infusions for wounds
54. Treating for when the head has been crushed and the brains are coming out
55. Ointments/salves

Here is the table of contents from the *Kihō:*

1. Stopping bleeding
2. Medicines that are to be imbibed internally
3. Infusions
4. Stopping aching
5. Moxibustion
6. The width of a wound
7. Making blood flow/run

8. Agada Powder [阿伽陀散]
9. Stopping pain within the body
10. Putting back in viscera
11. Knowing the depth of a wound
12. Bruise wounds
13. Treatment for when the mouth of the wound has dried [i.e., is not moist]
14. So that a wound will not become swollen
15. Treating the pain of a wound
16. Extracting a lodged arrowhead
17. Treating to dry the wound
18. Treatment for wounds to the eye from an arrow
19. Healing medicines for wounds
20. Treating for when the eyes do not see
21. Putting back in brains that are protruding from the head
22. Treating with *candock*
23. Treating smashed bones
24. The second initiation, by medicine
25. Not causing scars from the wound
26. The mouth of a wound becoming weepy
27. Constipation resulting from the injury
28. Treating deep cuts
29. Treating bones that have been cut
30. Treating wounds that have become swollen
31. Treating old wounds where the person has damaged what had been repaired
32. Reducing where the mouth of a wound has become raised
33. Wounds [suffered] when being drunk on rice wine
34. Treating wounds from being bitten by a wild boar or a deer
35. Seeing whether someone is dead or alive
36. Repairing sinews that have been cut
37. Seven Medicine compound
38. Black Medicine [黒薬]
39. Green Medicine [青薬]
40. White Medicine [白薬]
41. Fragrance medicines
42. Compounding Five Fragrances Infusion
43. Treating the wounds

This highly detailed delineation is far more comprehensive than that appearing in Chinese works and certainly more fulsome than what we find in Shōzen's writings. However, where did the knowledge come from? That is, what elements came together to produce a new field? And did Song medicine play a role in this?

New Sources of Knowledge: Human and Textual

The author of the *Kinsō ryōjishō* notes in the postscript that the work was based upon information about medicines and treatments that he had gained since the early 1330s and that he was prompted to write it down in order to facilitate treatment for hundreds of people wounded in battles in (it appears) the early 1350s. In the preface, the author notes two sources of his information. First, he met with twenty-eight noted physicians, asked them their secrets 口訣, and later collated the information and wrote it down. Second, he also examined Japanese and Chinese medical works 和漢医書 and then recorded the essentials. Together, he tells us, these constitute the overall lore 故実 of medicine and should be kept secret.[51] The author of *Kihō* notes that he has recorded the lore and the bulk of the oral transmissions 口伝 of wound physicians (which should not be shown to outsiders and should be kept secret).[52] However, he makes no mention of medical texts. Let us look in turn at these two elements, human and textual.

Prior to the 1330s, we have very little knowledge of people and places active in medicine outside of more learned circles. References to lineages or traditions are likewise sparse: As far as I am aware, the only such reference is that provided by Shōzen, who in the *Ton'ishō* notes a secret oral transmission for Joy Medicine 歡喜薬 in which the juice from the fruit of a certain tree is used as a lubricant to enhance sexual congress, is not to be transmitted to anyone for any amount of money, and is only known by six students of the Kawatsū Lay Priest (i.e., the warrior Itō Sukechika, d. 1182).[53]

By contrast, the wound texts are comparatively replete with names of people and places, and they refer to lineages of teaching. It might be that we learn of these simply because the author wrote them down, and that the lineages at least predate the 1330s. This might be particularly the case with those enmeshed in Buddhist networks, such as the anonymous late-Kamakura Nara priest whose healing repertoire did include a formula for treating wounds.[54] The most overt evidence of a Buddhist network appears in the *Kihō,* which refers many times to the oral transmissions of the Great Teacher of Mt. Kōya, the site of one of the major centers of Japanese esoteric Buddhism, and a title that brings to mind older traditions of secret knowledge associated with Buddhist ascetics.

The teachings of the Great Teacher are mentioned at least ten times, and they deal with such issues as a special added ingredient for medicine, preventing the spirit from going awry, when to apply moxibustion to a wound, medicine so that the condition of the body won't worsen, stopping the pain of the wound, preventing a wound swelling or getting cold, helping the wound to dry out, and ensuring that the wound heals quickly. The Great Teacher is also the source of two special "initiations," the first dealing with treatment for arms and legs that have been nearly cut off, and the second being knowledge of an evidently potent healing drink.[55] The Great Teacher also helps one determine whether a wound is fatal: "The transmission of the Great Teacher is: When looking to see whether the person will live or die, firstly, when one has [the person] drink life-preserving medicine 不死ノ薬, if it is regurgitated, [the person] will die; if it is not returned, [he] will live."[56]

But it is also possible that at least some lineages and individuals are mentioned because they only emerged in response to the sudden need for expertise in this field and that they and their medicines had gained some distinction. *Kihō* refers to oral transmissions of "myself" and others,[57] as well as to the transmission of the "demon formulas," from which the text apparently takes its name.[58] It also notes that knowledge of Twelve-Ingredient Green Medicine 十二青薬 should not transmitted without reason, since it is not known in any lineages apart from that of one Shichirō "Boat-Captain" Funagashira.[59] *Kinsō ryōjishō* is even more informative. We learn of a transmission from the Secret Store of the Tōtōmi Lay Priest, of the Yamato Sugimoto 大和杦本 ointment, a recipe from the Secret Store of one Uritsu no kan,[60] and of the Give-Five General, the Nanfu Lay Priest (who appears several times), or one Kakujō.[61] One location—Nonomura in the Yuji estate in Ōmi Province 近江之国湯次庄野村秘蔵—is mentioned several times and is noted for having a secret store of medicine.[62]

The second new source of knowledge was textual, at least in the case of the *Kinsō ryōjishō,* since the *Kihō* notes none at all. However, although the author of the *Kinsō ryōjishō* mentions that he had consulted Japanese and Chinese texts, unfortunately he only mentions two by name. One of them (noted in section 3) is a formula for stopping bleeding attributed to the *Qianjin fang*. The other reference is to the *Sanying fang* and appears in the preface where the author explicates the field of wound medicine. This reference seems to have provided the field of wound medicine with its conceptual basis.

The major theoretical contribution of the *Sanyin fang* to Song medicine, at least as understood in Japan, was its classification of the causes of injuries into three types. The first type was inner causes, whereby the disordered state of one's qi (which could be caused by one's emotional state) and of yin and yang in the body is manifested in damages to the internal organs. The second type was external causes, whereby ailments were produced by wind, cold, summer heat, dampness, dryness, and heat, which damage the skin and produce ailments. The third type, and relevant to wound medicine, was causes that were neither internal nor external and were produced by trauma injury unrelated to the prior state of the person's body, such as injuries from weapons, falls, fire, or animals. Apart from the obvious symptoms that could result from such injuries, the understanding of the nature of the injury was relevant for treatment for other problems resulting from the injury, such as delirium or fever.

This third type, "not inner or outer cause" 不内外因 (Ja. *fu naigai in*), was already known in Japan. However, it appears that this nosology had not initially been associated with wound medicine. As we have seen, Kajiwara Shōzen was well acquainted with the *Sanyin fang* and referred to its new nosology during his discussion of "all forms of [disorders of] qi."[63] Yet, strikingly, when talking about incised injury in the *Man'anpō,* Shōzen makes absolutely no reference to or cites any formulas from the *Sanyin fang,* even though he cites other Song works. And, evidently guided by the structure of the *Shengji zonglu* (which was compiled prior to the *Sanyin fang*), he gives no indication that he thought that the *Sanyin fang*'s "not inner or outer cause" might augment or supersede the *Shengji zonglu.* This is somewhat puzzling, but we may take it as further confirmation that when writing about wound medicine, Shōzen was not responding to any particular need for better conceptual understanding (beyond clarifying that it was a distinct medical category).

Thus, the fact that the author of *Kinsō ryōjishō* specifies that the conceptual basis for the treatment of wounds is different from that required to treat conditions of the body otherwise is a significant advance. As he notes in the preface to the *Kinsō ryōjishō*,

> First and foremost, what one should understand about wounds is what is stated in the *Sanyin fang.* Things that arise from the Six Bowels are called ailments from internal causes. Things that arise from the Five Viscera are called external ailments. Ailments that do not arise from the Six Bowels and Five Viscera are ailments that do not have internal or external causes. For example, ailments of the liver are manifested in the eye. Ailments of the lungs are manifested in the nose. But wounds are unrelated to any viscera. If there is any damage it is because it is an ailment that has no internal or external cause. Thus even if there is an injury to the eye, this is unrelated to any damage to the liver. If there is an injury to the nose, this is unrelated to any damage to the lungs.

However, it is not clear whether the author actually saw a copy of the *Sanyin fang* or had the information that it contains conveyed to him orally. In the *Kinsō ryōjishō,* the key phrase "not inner or outer cause" is miswritten. The "not" character, *fu* 不, is replaced with a homophone, the character for "government office," *fu* 府 (which character was itself a common rebus for "bowels," *fu* 腑), making the third category "government office (bowels) inner and outer cause," 府[腑]内外因. Perhaps the author, as noted, heard about the idea secondhand, relied upon an inaccurate copy (which would have to be a handwritten copy of a printed original), or made an error in transcription. We note an example of this in the reference to the medicine Divine Chinese-Angelica Ointment, which is transcribed as 神物當飾高 instead of 神物當皈[帰]膏 (parenthetically, the reader may recall the Divine Efficacy Chinese-Angelica Ointment formula from the *Ton'ishō* that was noted earlier). On the other hand, and far more likely, since the characters 府内外因 obviously make no sense in this context, it may have been a deliberate substitution that would be understood by those "in the know." In any event, whatever the immediate source of the author's knowledge of the *Sanyin fang,* he knew the title and understood the relevance of one of its key concepts for the treatment of wounds.

Notwithstanding the key role of the *Sanyin fang* in providing a conceptual basis for wound medicine, what might account for the lack of reference to other written texts, despite the fact that the author mentions that he had read some? My answer is necessarily speculative, but a few possibilities suggest themselves.

First, while the *Sanyin fang* provides a clear conceptual basis for understanding wound injury, the injuries do not present an etiological problem. There is no doubt as to what caused the trauma: falls; a cut or a slice from a blade; a puncture from a spear, arrow, stick, or bite; a break or crush from rocks, clubs, or heavy objects; one can also include burns and scalds from fire and hot liquid, frostbite, and insect and animal bites. Moreover, unlike an issue such as *rai* leprosy, there were no religious or moral issues surrounding wound injury that would require substantial theoretical engagement.

Second, a number of practical concerns may have limited the utility of any information in written Song works. For one thing, while books are portable, it may not have been feasible to carry them around and consult them. For another, extrapolating from Shōzen's comment that most physicians did not read formula handbooks and the fact that he wrote the *Ton'ishō* in Japanese so that the medical knowledge would be better disseminated, it is possible that few physicians would have been literate enough to understand written Chinese. Another element may have been that information about wound medicine in Chinese texts varied, naturally reflecting the purpose for which a work was written. Many formula manuals do not address the topic in any useful depth; the *Yeshi luyan fang,* for example, has little more than a few lines on incised wounds.[64] And as far as I am aware, Chinese works known to have been available in Japan do not provide useful information on the range of issues that, as we can see from the indices to the *Kinsō ryōjishō* and the *Kihō,* actually confronted physicians treating trauma injury. A final point may be that texts may not have provided useful information on treating certain types of injuries that may have been more common in Japan because of Japanese weapons and ways in warfare. The case need not be overstated, since warfare anywhere can generate a range of injuries. But one should at least be aware, for example, that Japanese arrowheads came in a "bewildering variety of shapes and sizes,"[65] and that the Japanese sword produces its own type of deep slashing wounds, thus requiring that people be particularly versed in ways to treat the resulting injuries.

In sum, the paucity of references to Song medical works in the first two wound medicine texts indicates that they might not have been particularly relevant sources of knowledge. That is to say, they might not have been able to provide better information on treating wounds than may already have been available to wound specialists. This, then, raises the question of from where wound medicine specialists may have gotten their knowledge.

Existing Sources of Knowledge

There being no known written guides to treating incised injury and apparently very few people with much expertise in the area, those treating battle injuries needed to extrapolate from what they already knew. Battlefield injuries typically involved particular types of injury (slashes and cuts, punctures, and the like) that were caused by certain sorts of weapons (blades, spears, arrows, and blunt objects). However, while one should not minimize the particularities of battle injury (such as an arrowhead lodged in bone), treatment of battle injury had much in common with treatment for a range of generic traumas that might be suffered in ordinary circumstances. These included bruising, swellings, burning and scalding by hot liquid (water or oil), weeping and pustulent wounds, the need to stop bleeding, internal organs either protruding or needing to be held in, fractured or broken bones, general abrasions, frostbite, and even insect and animal bites. In addition and as noted in wound medicine texts, the injured needed to be treated for pain, shock, delirium, lack of appetite, and constipation or diarrhea, and they required help with recuperation and restoration of their overall constitution.

While the wound injury specialists have left us no hint as to their knowledge base, it is possible to obtain some sense of what it might have been from the *Ton'ishō*. As is known, the *Ton'ishō* was directed to a general audience. I will not claim that all wound specialists would have been directly familiar with the formulas noted but rather that they are a guide to contemporary medical concerns. What is quite striking is that a considerable amount of information relevant to the treatment of battle injury derives from the treatment of women's medical needs, which were in the normal course of events accorded much attention.

With respect to the treatment of swellings, chapter 21 (on pains in the abdominal and genitourinary regions) prescribes a secret Black Medicine for a scrotum that is swollen or hard, and another secret, unnamed medicine for bringing down the swelling.[66] Chapter 29 (one of the seven chapters devoted to women's medicine) has a number of formulas, often involving daubing afflicted areas with liquid applications, for treating such concerns as when the area to the left and right of the vagina is swollen, the skin inflamed, and the itching and pain unbearable. In one case, the formula is also recommended for treating a swollen penis.[67] On a different topic, treatment for flesh that has been torn, chapter 29 gives a number of formulas for dealing with tears and wounds suffered by women as a result of sexual intercourse (literally, "having been opened by a man"),[68] while chapter 33 (mainly postpartum problems) contains formulas for conditions such as vaginal (perineal?) tearing; the labia/vulva extruded, swollen, torn, and "not coming back together"; and an extruded and torn vagina.[69]

For dealing with damaged flesh, chapter 24 (covering boils, carbuncles, and the like) provides much information. One formula, Transform the Poison Expel the Pus Inner Augmenting Powder 化毒排膿内補散, combines a secret Black Medicine that is to be drunk throughout the period of treatment with a special ointment. The ointment is to be applied on top of the red, swollen, and pustulent site; the bad flesh, if rotten or putrefied and not too painful, should all be cut away; when the swelling has gone down and matter issues from the bottom of the sore, the spot is to be washed once every two or three days with water in which lotus leaf and Asian plantain have been boiled and the ointment reapplied. And, reflecting beliefs that the efficacy of the medicine might be diminished by baleful influences (beliefs also noted earlier in the treatment of *rai*), Shōzen notes that a pregnant woman who is drinking it must not look at a menstruating woman nor at a person with physical disabilities, and she must not draw close to people wearing red clothing.[70] At least two other special medicines are mentioned. One is an unnamed secret medicine that successfully treats all thirteen types of carbuncles and requires the utilization of different parts of the plant depending upon the season.[71] Another medicine, Cloud Mother (Mica) Ointment 雲母膏, was comprised of no fewer than forty ingredients and was recommended for all types of boils, swellings, cuts, or breaks, and it is claimed that, provided wind had not been drawn into the wound, once applied there will be no further damage to the area for the following thirty years.[72]

The *Ton'ishō* also devotes considerable attention to the question of bleeding (that is, how to stop it). Chapter 23, "Various Bleeding Conditions," offers a number of formulas for treating such things as bloody stools and bloody urine, vomiting blood, nosebleeds, bleeding hemorrhoids, bleeding from the throat, and bleeding and injury to the five viscera as a result of falling from a horse or a high place.[73] Chapter 27 gives the formula for a secret medicine for dealing with menstruation that does not cease or for postpartum bleeding.[74] Chapter 29 provides formulas for dealing with blood in the urine or bleeding from the nose.[75] Chapter 31 has formulas for treating unceasing bleeding following a miscarriage and discusses as well what to do when a pregnant woman's stomach is painful and she is producing pustulent blood.[76] Finally, chapter 32 takes up postpartum bleeding that does not stop.[77]

Extrusions are another relevant subject. For treating a protruding vagina (prolapsed uterus?), chapter 29 gives a formula that involves applying charred turtle head mixed with water. Another treatment recommends combining a medicinal brew and the charred leaves of the white oak tree, applying it with one hand and pushing on the extruding part; "then it will without fail go in."[78] Chapter 33 has treatments, such as Sulfur Powder 硫黄散 or Jade Dragon Decoction 玉龍湯, for postpartum vaginal (uterine?) prolapse and tearing.[79] Chapter 36, one of five pediatric chapters, has a number of treatments (many from the *Hejiju fang*) for infant prolapsed anus, such as prolapsed anus due to diarrhea or cold in the abdomen, for which one daubs a treatment on the protrusion and pushes it back in.[80]

Easing pain is another concern. In chapter 21 are found formulas, many taken from the *Sanyin fang,* for alleviating such things as sudden and unbearable pelvic and genital pain, stabbing pain, and a pain that is so bad that the person wants to die. One formula, Twin-Purpose Gold Pill 兼金円, is prescribed for pain in the stomach, and it is also recommended for pains accompanying menstruation.[81] On a similar topic, chapter 27 gives a secret remedy for treating severe pains that occur during menstruation.[82] Chapter 29 provides a number of formulas for postpartum pain and the formula Alum Powder 白礬散 for pain caused by vaginal swelling (for which a suppository, to be changed two to three times daily, is employed).[83] Chapter 32 provides an additional formula for dealing with unbearable postpartum stomach pain, another for unceasing pain, and a number of unnamed formulas for treating postpartum dizziness and delirium.[84]

These various concerns are, to reiterate, ones with which the wound medicine texts deal. The suggestion that generic knowledge was utilized by and applied to wound medicine draws additional support from the fact that, conversely, the wound medicine texts also sometimes note when formulas for wound medicine might be applied to other areas. For example, section 44 of *Kinsō ryōjishō* notes that a medicine to be ingested for wounds is likewise good for treating falls from a horse, carriage, or high place. Section 12 of *Kihō,* which deals with bruise wounds, likewise contains formulas that the author recommends in the treatment of fractures and breaks incurred as a result of falling from a high place or from a horse. Section 41 of *Kihō* notes that Fragrance Medicines, one of which is a "secret transmission" containing thirty-three ingredients, are good for all types of swellings. The author notes that another one is also particularly effective for treating sores and carbuncles.[85] And in section 43 of *Kihō,* we find the comment that Warm White Pill 温白丸, which is the prime purgative medicine in the Secret Store, is also a secret medicine for the treatment of Mountain Ailment (that is, *rai* leprosy). Warm White Pill is said to be miraculously effective when treating skin and flesh that is peeling off, though when treating wounds a lesser dose is recommended.

These texts also confirm that physicians readily identified parallels in the treatment of wounds and the treatment of women's medical problems. Section 44 of *Kinsō ryōjishō*—the topic of which is (ingested) medicine for wounds—observes, for example, that Japan White Medicine 日本白薬 is also good for treating women's postpartum delirium. Section 40 of *Kihō* similarly remarks that Japan White Medicine is efficacious for postpartum delirium due to the afterbirth's not being expelled. Section 7 of *Kihō* recommends that medicine for purging blood may be used not only in the case of wounds but also for blood wellings during pregnancy and childbirth. Section 27 on constipation resulting from injury includes an entry noting that fresh Rehmannia is good for constipation resulting from both wounds and childbirth.

In sum, the information required for treating battle injury most likely came from existing sources of medical knowledge within Japan. It is not impossible that information on treatments for wound injury that derived from Song sources found its way indirectly into wound medicine texts via information contained in Shōzen's work and disseminated through known Buddhist networks. Nonetheless, it probably makes more sense to assume that, in the circumstances of the time, this would have been overall quite limited.

However, when one shifts attention to the materia medica used in the treatment of wound injury, there is somewhat more evidence of Song medicine.

MATERIA MEDICA AND SONG MEDICINE

The wound medicine texts mention some 130 items of materia medica, which we can divide into materials originating from plants, animals, and minerals, and items otherwise prepared for human consumption (such as rice wine). The overwhelming majority of these are of indigenous origin. But we also find at least twenty-six that are of overseas origin. Most are readily identifiable as such: cardamom, Dragon's Blood, cloves, cassia, Burmese rosewood, white sandalwood, aloes, Chinese licorice, turmeric, ginseng, Borneo camphor tree, fennel, frankincense, chebulic myrobalan, ginger, croton, betel nut, musk, rhinoceros horn, tiger bones, and fossil bones 竜骨 *(Os draconis)*. In six other cases, the authors specify that the item must be of the Chinese variety: Chinese sesame, Chinese bamboo, Chinese costus, Chinese fern, Chinese millet, and Chinese mugwort.[86]

Noted earlier (see chapter 3) was that the demands of warfare stimulated the demand for overseas materia medica, but here I want to make a different point: Namely, even though the city of Kamakura was no longer a major center of consumption, overseas trade continued to be funneled through Hakata and warfare seems not to have interrupted the circulation of goods. To the contrary, warfare in the fourteenth century opened up new opportunities for trade and commerce. Thus, items of overseas materia medica that were integral to Song formulas were familiar and readily available. Moreover, given that there were probably few written guides to these, one can perhaps state the obvious and note that they became known through word of mouth. Thus, even if, as will be seen, wound physicians did not use what can be readily identified as specific formulas drawn from Song medicine, they were beneficiaries of the Song pharmaceutical regime.

Sometimes the overseas item is only one among many ingredients, as with a formula from the *Kihō* for treating swollen cuts: "Medicine for packing a swelling caused by a cut: ash of an edible river shell, ash of oyster [shell], ash of clam [shell], powder of Burmese rosewood, ash of a human bregma [天盖[蓋]], deer antler, and roasted salt; adding vinegar to rice paste, make a watery glutinate, then mix with equal portions of the ashes, smear paper with it, and apply it above the swelling."[87]

More often than not, however, these overseas items seem to have been seen as having particularly potent healing properties, and they often appear alongside other such ingredients in formulas for treating some of the more challenging injuries. For example, for mending bones that have been cut, *Kinsō ryōjishō* prescribes as follows:

> If the shin or the arm has been deeply cut or sliced, even though one night may have passed and even if the person rendering aid is late, put willow wood that has been wrapped in a boiling cloth into hot water and steam it. Place the cut section of what has been cut above this and warm it up [with the hot vapors], and [then] shave Dragon's Blood resin into the marrow of the bone. Stand a ready stalk in this and apply it. Tiger's Bones are also good. If you do not have either of these [resin or Tiger's Bones], you should shave a [dried] umbilical cord and apply it. In the case of males, the umbilical cord of a female child is best.[88]

Overseas materia medica were also used in a niche area: fragrance medicines. Given that *Kihō* lists three versions of one of them, Five Fragrances Infusion 五香煎, the same infusion that was introduced some 150 years earlier by Eisai in his *Kissa Yōjōki,* one might conclude that they were quite popular. Perhaps the best example of a successful fragrance medicine is the unnamed formula that is a secret transmission and the compounding of which takes three days and three nights. Recommended as excellent for swellings rather than wounds, it contains no fewer than thirty-three ingredients, at least fifteen of which are imported materia medica.[89] Clearly, this is further firm evidence that the type of formula that we have identified as derived from Islamic medicine and which became a part of Song medicine had not only been transmitted to Japan, but was likely in widespread use.

CONCLUDING COMMENTS

The emergence of wound medicine as a medical specialty in the fourteenth century was directly related to the unanticipated outbreak of endemic warfare. While there was some knowledge of how to treat battle injury and traumas in general, even someone as well read and with as much clinical experience as Kajiwara Shōzen had not paid it particular attention. We need not see this as a particular failing of medicine in a society at peace, but it did mean that detailed knowledge about medicines and treatment had to be gained essentially on the job.

In gaining their experience, physicians did not look to written medical works but rather extrapolated from generic knowledge that could be applied to the treatment of wounds. While there are questions about whether the level of literacy of most physicians would have been sufficient to understand Chinese medical works, it also seems that the information on the treatment of wounds contained in those Chinese works that we know to have been available may not have been particularly helpful—or demonstrably better. Also—while I have not dwelt on these factors—the fluid dynamics of warfare and the basic absence of logistic or support services for warriors meant that books might not have been accorded great priority.

Nonetheless, Song medicine did contribute substantially to the development of wound medicine in Japan in two ways. First, Japanese physicians made use of items of materia medica that had become available through increased trade with China and that had become familiar because they were essential ingredients in the Song formulas that had been adopted during the Kamakura period. That is, the Song pharmaceutical ecology had been transferred to Japan and become domesticated. Second, while Song medicine did not provide much technical knowledge about wound medicine, it did, courtesy of the *Sanyin fang,* provide a conceptual basis for wound medicine where one did not exist before. Moreover, the conceptual basis was clear and no doubt could be readily understood. As such, Song medicine provided wound medicine—which developed as the quintessential medical specialty of the medieval era—with important grounding.

Epilogue

ENGAGING SONG MEDICAL KNOWLEDGE

The preceding chapters have taken up several topics relating to the acquisition of medical writings, the engagement of a new pharmaceutical regime, and some reasons for and ways in which new information was understood and integrated. Here I would like to make a number of broader observations relating to the appropriation, testing, and refining of medical knowledge. While it is generally known that in the premodern era Japanese physicians—and indeed specialists in many areas—engaged new knowledge and sought ways to utilize it, little attention has been paid to the actual processes involved. It is hoped that the following remarks, which will focus on Shōzen, will serve at least as an introduction to these matters.

I will divide my comments into three areas. First I will comment on some issues related to the transmission and appropriation of book knowledge and some of the things that Shōzen gained from Song medicine. Second, I will comment on issues relevant to the clinical engagement of that new knowledge and shed some light on the process of inquiry. Third, I will touch on the interaction of different systems of explanation, what I broadly characterize as Buddhist and Chinese. I will cite one example where Song-era Chinese medicine was confirmed by reference to a Buddhist understanding and another example where Buddhist understanding was superseded by a Chinese understanding.

ISSUES OF TRANSMISSION AND APPROPRIATION OF BOOK KNOWLEDGE

An essential prerequisite for learning about Song Chinese medical knowledge was having some idea of what works were available—and then, of course, having access to a collection housing these physical items. We need not assume that Shōzen, or indeed anyone else for that matter, would have known the entire universe of works from which selection might be made. But there is little doubt that collection development in Japan in this time represented a substantial advance over such earlier bibliographic collection endeavors. The range of items available was broader. Thanks to the Song print revolution, they were more readily available than at any previous time. The contact with China was continuous rather than sporadic, making access and acquisition an essentially standard process. There were also multiple routes by which the material might make its way to Japan: trips sponsored by political authority or by individual temples, maritime traders, Chinese coming to Japan, or Japanese who had sojourned in China.

Yet amid the regularity, one might usefully recognize that serendipity played a part. There seems to have been no master catalog of works available in China. While some works may have been particularly desirable (such as texts central to religious traditions or well-known encyclopedic or medical works), there is no evidence of a sustained and targeted acquisition program. Since Shōzen never went to China himself, it might reasonably be assumed that the landscape of Song medical knowledge was created by others for him, albeit with the best of intentions to supply him with works that would in sum be current, useful, and comprehensive. The selection of titles also likely reflected different factors, such as the recommendation of a physician in China, physical availability in a southern Chinese bookstore, that the person acquiring them knew that a work was well regarded or might be useful in Kamakura, or that the acquirer was aware that people in Japan were interested in getting Chinese medical works. But lest we jump to the conclusion that the acquisition process was simply random, it is useful to bear in mind that relying upon a web of contacts and routes does not seem to be an unusual way to assemble a collection. And, in Shōzen's case, the result was access to contemporary medical works of great quality and breadth.

We have very few examples from the premodern era where we can move beyond simply noting that a work or some works had been acquired and see how the information was actually utilized. Shōzen thus provides us with a useful window into the process of the appropriation of knowledge. His citation of sources, the manner in which he assembled the information into his chapters, his comments on various theories about illness, his suggestions about adjusting formulas or ingredients, and his reflections on the discoveries that he was making all tell us what information he drew from which works and what he was learning from them. It might of course be pointed out that our information would be more complete if, apart from those instances where he notes the failings of current practices or previous knowledge, Shōzen had commented on why he did not, for example, select a formula for inclusion. On the other hand, perhaps the lack of a working commentary in a finished compilation need not detract from the larger points.

We are also able to discover what Shōzen specifically may have learned about the field of medicine itself, which stands in contrast to what had characterized Japanese medicine to that point. Shōzen realized that, while concerns about proprietary knowledge remained, medicine was a fairly public endeavor rather than a closed enterprise. Medicine was also an extensive branch of knowledge that was inhabited by a variety of specialty areas and fields that produced their own works and generated their own inquiries. Medicine was a dynamic enterprise in which understanding evolved. While it remained important to transmit understandings and to organize and systematize knowledge, it was also important to avoid ossification and to be receptive to new interpretations and formulas.

CLINICAL ENGAGEMENT AND THE PROCESS OF INQUIRY

Shōzen had access to a substantial number of medical works that encapsulated significant new understandings of illness. Those works also provided Shōzen with at least 25,000 formulas from which he might select ones for clinical examination and from which he selected the overwhelming bulk of the 1,400 formulas included the *Ton'ishō* and the 3,100 formulas included in the *Man'anpō.* The formulas included a substantial range of new materia medica made available via the extensive Pharmaceutical Silk Road, and they embodied the substantial changes in the Chinese pharmaceutical regime that had shaped Song medicine. Japanese knowledge of the Chinese pharmaceutical regime was lagging by several centuries, so the formulas and materia medica provided a qualitative leap forward for Japanese medicine.

Yet this new knowledge needed first to be understood and interpreted. That is, while the information may have been prepackaged, it needed to be unwrapped before it became useful. No doubt understanding the Chinese pharmacopoeia and making professional judgments about writings and formulas posed a challenge even for Chinese physicians. But Shōzen faced a steep learning curve that required precise, long-term attention, and his engagement provides us a sense of the process of scientific inquiry that was entailed. Technical translation, without which the absorption or appropriation of new knowledge could not proceed, was central. Shōzen understood that the Song pharmacopoeia was substantially different from the Tang pharmacopoeia, and the Japanese knowledge base for understanding the Chinese pharmacopoeia was no longer adequate. Updating it required comparison of variant nomenclatures and clarification of the accuracy and provenance of the units of measurement in formulas. Experimentation with amounts of the ingredients was required so that a formula might become a useful prescription. It was also necessary to understand the materia medica. Many items were new and not native to Japan. It also became apparent that some earlier Japanese identifications were incorrect, requiring apparently detailed cross-checking of Song information with existing Japanese reference material, such as the *Honzō wamyō* (Japanese Handbook of Materia Medica). It is not known whether Shōzen from the outset determined to compare the older information with the new or simply came to realize that there were enough discrepancies to make him question the overall accuracy of the centuries-old knowledge. His efforts, as far as we can tell, involved meticulous testing, analysis, reformulation, winnowing, and comparison.

A further sense of the process of inquiry is obtained from the responses to two pressing contemporary social and medical issues: *rai* and wound medicine. Neither *rai* nor trauma injury was a new phenomenon, but both presented a substantial medical challenge. *Rai* was arguably the greater challenge, since the etiology of the affliction was unknown, physicians entertained different explanations about the cause, it required treatment over an extended period of time with no certainty that the affliction might be ameliorated, and those afflicted or determined to be afflicted with it were liable to be stigmatized and shunned. By contrast, the causes of traumatic wound injury were quite obvious.

On the other hand, both *rai* and wound injury shared commonalities. In a longer-term context whereby medicine had largely involved treating internal constitutional imbalance and the medicines that were prescribed were essentially ones that were ingested, these two clinical challenges focused attention on traumas on the surface of the body. While we may be fairly certain that not all treatments would be efficacious from a modern medical standpoint, we might also feel confident that physicians were able to discern what treatments might not be particularly useful. After all, physicians in both areas would have had ample opportunity to learn what treatments simply were not having much effect and discard them in favor of ones that—if not perhaps solving all problems—were at least understood as better.

DIFFERENT SYSTEMS OF EXPLANATION

Shōzen was heir to at least two broadly defined lineages of medical epistemology or disease etiology. The first was the Buddhist and the second was the Chinese. With respect to the former, early Indian Buddhist injunctions regarding compassion, the doing of good works, the importance of tending to the medical needs of the monastic community, and the central nature of the Healing Buddha combined to shape a homologized Buddhist medical system. Prayer, magic, and medicinals coexisted, each element recognized as integral, and no one element seems to have been privileged over the others.[1] With respect to the Chinese lineage, while it too encompassed magical medicine, and charms and chants played a part in healing, the early development of highly sophisticated systems of classification of pharmaceuticals and ailments and ongoing efforts by physicians and theorists to refine understandings suggest that, as a comparative matter, the Chinese lineage placed more emphasis on pharmaceuticals and on the development of medicines.

Both lineages came to Japan via China. Whatever actual interactions may have occurred in Chinese context, they were initially transmitted to Japan as separate entities and housed in separate institutional settings. We do not have sufficient information to know whether aristocratic court physicians, the recipients of Tang medical knowledge, had any knowledge of Buddhist disease etiology or even whether they would have had access to Buddhist texts that touched on healing. Most likely, they did not. Conversely, we do not have any information on whether Buddhist priests who were physicians in their monastic community would have had much knowledge of Chinese medicine or much access to Chinese medical texts (apart perhaps from some pharmacological works). Priest-physicians also likely did not have access to Buddhist texts on healing through ritual and prayer that were the province of esoteric specialists.

While there is much that is unknown about Shōzen's life, however, he seems not to have had much investment in the Heian structure of medical knowledge that these traditions represented. He belonged to a new Kamakura-era sect that was building its own traditions, which looked to Song Chinese sources for texts and models, and which was directly engaged in providing medical treatment. Accordingly, it would be a mistake to see Shōzen as heir to either specific Buddhist medical traditions that existed in Japan or to the learned traditions of Japanese court medicine. Like his sect, Shōzen represented a break with—or at least an orientation away from—past practices, rather than continuity with them. And if we do place him in a lineage, then it is the Buddhist one that placed emphasis on healing through materia medica rather than through ritual. In any event, Shōzen was open to evaluating different theories of illness and was not wedded to inherited knowledge. Two examples illustrate this fact.

The first example relates to Shōzen's observation that Buddhism and Chinese medicine share a common view that ultimately all illnesses originate in the mind, in the context of Shōzen's effort to understand the new Song disease category of "all forms of [disorders of] qi," which had been classified in the *Sanyin fang* as disorders arising from "internal causes." Shōzen, in seeking to absorb the perspective that such ailments were the product of the seven qi, drew an explicit connection with the basic Buddhist understanding that mind is the root of all problems. In short, Shōzen was able to grasp the validity of a new understanding in Chinese medicine because it could be confirmed by Buddhist teaching.

The second example likewise involves an assessment of the validity of Buddhist and Chinese explanations—but with a different outcome. Both Buddhist and Chinese medicine wrestled with how to explain some ailments that were difficult to cure (*rai* leprosy, corpse-transmitted diseases) or that were congenital. The Buddhist default explanation was the notion of karma, which at least some medieval Japanese equated with the Chinese idea of destiny. That this understanding was not inaccurate is confirmed in the Song work *Rencun Sunshi zhibing huofa mifang,* in which the issue of what specifically causes corpse-transmitted disease (worms) is posed separately from the question of why one person rather than another might contract the affliction (karma, destiny, legacy of ancestors). As a medical issue, however, Rencun's explanation that worms were to blame was more useful to Shōzen.

For Shōzen, the major explanatory challenge involving karma related to *rai*. Shōzen's clinical experience led him to understand that *rai* was not necessarily karmic in nature and that the number of *rai* that were understood as karmic might diminish if effective treatment was found. This led to him to accept that a Song medical explanation was a superior model for an affliction that had been previously understood in terms of basic Buddhist textual teaching. Since the notion of karma is so fundamental to Buddhism, at first glance this appears surprising. However, it is entirely possible that another Buddhist perspective—that truths are relative and explanations are expedient devices subject to change—may have facilitated this shift in favor of Song knowledge.

ABBREVIATIONS

The following abbreviations are used in the notes and in the bibliography. Each work has an entry in the bibliography.

CHSS	*Chūsei hōsei shiryō shū*
GR	*Gunsho ruijū*
KI	*Kamakura ibun komonjo hen*
KT	*Kokushi taikei*
NBI-Ch	*Nanbokuchō ibun Chūgoku Shikoku hen*
NBI-Ka	*Nanbokuchō ibun Kantō hen*
NBI-Ky	*Nanbokuchō ibun Kyūshū hen*
NBI-To	*Nanbokuchō ibun Tōhoku hen*
NKBT	*Nihon koten bungaku taikei*
T	*Taishō shinshū Daizōkyō*
WND	*Writings of Nichiren Daishōnin*
ZGR	*Zoku Gunsho ruijū*

NOTES

Introduction

1. For the few studies of Shōzen's life and work, see Ishihara Akira, "Kajiwara Shōzen no shōgai to sono chosho"; Hattori Toshirō, *Kamakura jidai igakushi no kenkyū,* pp. 93–158; Yamada Shigemasa, "Kajiwara Shōzen to sono shūi"; Adachihara Akiko, "*Man'anpō* shōnimon ni mirareru *Shōkanron* no eikyō"; and Adachihara Akiko, "*Man'anpō* no shōnimon ni tsuite."
2. I have used two editions of the *Ton'ishō:* first, an unpaginated microfilm hard copy of a text from the Naikaku Bunko, held in the Department of Medical History of the Oriental Medicine Research Institute of the Kitasato Institute, to which I make chapter references; second, in my citations I also make references to the Kagaku Shoin facsimile edition, which may be more readily available. However, whereas the former is clear and legible throughout, the legibility and readability of the latter vary considerably from chapter to chapter. This edition is also compiled of selections from different manuscripts. It is not a preferred reference tool, but it does allow more precise references.
3. For the *Man'anpō,* I have primarily used the 1986 Kagaku Shoin facsimile edition, and this is the source I cite in notes. I have also utilized but do not cite as such an unpaginated microfilm hard copy of a text held in the Department of Medical History of the Oriental Medicine Research Institute of the Kitasato Institute.
4. This translation supersedes my earlier version of the title, "Essentials of Medicine." Two useful editions of *Ishinpō* are *Nihon igaku sōsho katsujibon* and *Zen'yaku seikai Ishinpō.* For two partial English translations, see C. H. Hsia, Ilza Veith, and Robert H. Geertsma, *The Essentials of Medicine in Ancient China and Japan: Yasuyori Tanba's Ishinpo;* Howard Levy and Ishihara Akira, *The Tao of Sex: An Annotated Translation of the Twenty-Eighth Section of the Essence of Medical Prescriptions (Ishinpo).* For an introduction

to the text and its transmission, see Sugitatsu Yoshikazu, *Ishinpō no denrai.* For a useful overview, see Shinmura Taku, *Nihon iryō shakaishi no kenkyū,* pp. 274–281.

5. For a more extensive discussion of this topic, see the introduction in Andrew Edmund Goble, Kenneth R. Robinson, and Haruko Wakabayashi, eds., *Tools of Culture: Japan's Cultural, Intellectual, Medical, and Technological Contacts in East Asia, 1000s to 1500s.*
6. For more detail, see Hattori Toshirō, *Kamakura jidai igakushi no kenkyū,* pp. 93–158.
7. *Ton'ishō,* chapter 8 (Kagaku Shoin edition, 1986, p. 177, section V, leaves 71-72). Hereafter, *Ton'ishō,* chapter 8 (*KS,* p. 177, V-71-72). This is also partially cited in Hattori Toshirō, *Kamakura jidai igakushi no kenkyū,* pp. 99, 104.

Chapter 1 The Kamakura Context

1. I thus depart from the chronology of overseas influence offered in David Swain and Masayoshi Sugimoto, *Science and Culture in Traditional Japan, A.D. 600–1854.* The authors suggest that an "Early Chinese Cultural Wave II" started in 1401, following on from "The Semi-Seclusion Era: 894–1401."
2. See Ivo Smits, "China as Classic Text: Chinese Books and Twelfth-Century Japanese Collectors." The *Taiping yulan* example is found on p. 197.
3. On Kyushu and foreign contacts, see Bruce Batten's definitive *Gateway to Japan: Hakata in War and Peace, 500–1300.*
4. Bruce Batten, "An Open and Shut Case? Thoughts on Late Heian Overseas Trade," p. 310.
5. Shinmura Taku, *Nihon iryō shakai shi no kenkyū,* p. 374, noting entries from the *Shōyūki* from Chōwa 3 (1014).6.25 and 6.28.
6. *Gyokuyō,* Kaō 2 (1170).9.20 (1.107).
7. *Heike monogatari,* book 3, chapter 11: Hiroshi Kitagawa and Bruce Tsuchida, *The Tale of the Heike,* pp. 193–197; Helen Craig McCullough, *The Tale of the Heike,* pp. 115–117.
8 See Ethan Segal, "Awash With Coins: The Spread of Money in Medieval Japan," pp. 341–345.
9. See Gu Wenbi and Lin Shimin, "Neiha ni genzon suru Nihon koku Dazaifu Hakata tsū no kakyō kokuseki no kenkyū," pp. 103–104, for the inscriptions.
10. Antei 2 (1228).3.13 Kantō gechijō (*Kamakura ibun komonjo hen,* vol. 6, document 3732; hereafter cited as *KI,* 6:3732).
11. *Gyokuyō,* Kenkyū 2 (1191).2.19 (3.661).

12. Ms. Zhang's family story as revealed in legal documents is a particularly poignant one, involving one of her sons murdering another son, commending land to relatives, her death on the journey back from a legal hearing while accompanied by her daughter, and her bitter last words that she would never forgive her murderous son. Her commendation of land to her mother-in-law Ms. Wang is recorded on a stone stele. See Saeki Kōji, *Mongoru shūrai no totsugeki,* p. 29 for a picture; for the text, see Jōkyū 2 (1220).2.12 Chōshi kishinjō (*KI,* 5:2576). For the larger family story, see Bun'ei 5 (1264).6.27 Kantō hikitsukeshū renshō hōsho (*KI,* 13:10266), Bun'ei 5 (1264).7.3 Shami Jōkei (Munakata Ujinari) ukebumi (*KI,* 13:10274), Bun'ei 6 (1265).2 Azukari dokoro kudashibumi (*KI,* 14:10390).
13. On Ennin, see Edwin O. Reischauer, *Ennin's Travels in Tang China,* and *Ennin's Diary: A Record of a Pilgrimage to China in Search of the Law.* On Jōjin, see Robert Borgen, "Jōjin's Discoveries in Song China," and "Jōjin's Travels from Center to Center (with Some Periphery in Between)."
14. For the text and useful discussions of *Kissa yōjōki,* see Furuta Shōkin, *Eisai Kissa yōjōki,* and Mori Shikazō, *Honzōgaku kenkyū,* pp. 342–489.
15. *Azuma kagami,* Kenpō 2 (1214).2.4.
16. Mori Shikazō, *Honzōgaku kenkyū,* pp. 448–449 and p. 446 note 46.
17. For the Kyushu physicians, see *Gyokuyō,* Angen 3 (Jishō 1, 1177).6.4 (2.52), 1177.6.10 (2.56), when the "Chinzei physician priest Kenshōbō" and the "Tsukushi physician priest Daizenbō" were brought in to treat *kakke;* both recommended moxibustion.
18. I have drawn on the definitive treatment of Xie Guoming, Kawazoe Shōji's "Jōtenji no kaisō to Hakata gōshū Sha Kokumei [Xie Guoming]: Kamakura chūki no taigai kankei to Hakata," and on Saeki Kōji, *Mongoru shūrai no totsugeki,* pp. 30–33. One measure of Guoming's importance is that we have a statue of him, which as far as I am aware is the only image of a Chinese person resident in Japan who was not a religious figure prior to at least the seventeenth century. For a photograph of the statue of Xie Guoming held in Jōtenji, see Nishioka Reizō and Yanagita Yoshitaka, *Genkō to Hakata: Shashin de yomu Mōko shūrai,* p. 19. We only have a limited sense of Guoming's property holdings. See the suit against Guoming's widow brought by Munakata Shrine seeking the return of lands: Kenchō 4 (1252).7.12 Kantō mikyōsho (*KI,* 10:7458) and Kenchō 5 (1253).5.3 Hōjō Nagatoki kakikudashi (*KI,* 10:7551).
19. See the *Fumon-in Kyō Ron Shō So Goroku Jusho ra mokuroku.* The medical works are listed on pp. 392–393. They are cataloged in four groups: eight titles in Jade 玉, seven in Egression 出, three in Kun Mountain 崑, and eleven in Hill 崗. The catalog is divided into fifty such named groups, but I am unclear as to the organizing principle—it may simply have been

what titles were in a "bundle." For the listing of the works, see also Kosoto, "Kansu bon kara Sōgen ban e," pp. 468–470.

20. For some sense of the Kujō library in the late 1200s, see 1293.6.17 Kujō ke bunko monjo mokuroku (*KI,* 23.18125).
21. Ueda Jun'ichi, "Tōfukuji to Saidaiji—jibyō Monjū shinkō wo megutte."
22. For an excellent survey, see Kenneth Zysk, *Asceticism and Healing in Ancient India.*
23. *Man'anpō,* chapter 52 (Kagaku Shoin edition, 1986, p. 1398, section LII, leaves 134-135). Hereafter cited as *Man'anpō* chapter 52 (*KS,* p. 1398, LII-134-135). For information on the medicine, see *Man'anpō* chapter 52 (*KS,* pp. 1397–1398, LII-130-135).
24. *Man'anpō,* chapter 22 (*KS* p. 621, XXII-79-80), where Shōzen has a glowing endorsement of the formula known as Longlife Medicine 長生薬. It treats all types of swellings and sores from the very first through to relief: "Just put it on the swollen spot and it brings down the swelling; it gets rid of toxicity and adjusts cold and heat; it is of miraculous efficacy without parallel. This formula was a secret theory of a Chinese person, and even though people know of this formula they are unaware of its origins. The Japanese priest Dōshō lived in China and had it transmitted to him."
25. Ishihara Akira, "Kajiwara Shōzen no shōgai to sono chosho," pp. 1741–1742; Ueda Jun'ichi, "Tōfukuji to Saidaiji: jibyō Monjū shinkō wo megutte;" Kojima Takayuki, "Mujū denki shokō: ijutsu to shisō wo megutte," pp. 44–45. For more on Mujū and a partial English translation of *Shasekishū,* see Robert E. Morrell, *Sand and Pebbles.* For a photograph of Chōboji and an Edo period map of the temple and its grounds, see Ōsumi Kazuo, *Shinshin no sekai, tonseisha no kokoro,* pp. 40–41.
26. Shinmura Taku, *Kodai iryō kanjin sei no kenkyū,* pp. 337–338. For Minji, see Kyotofu Ishikai, ed., *Kyoto no igakushi,* p. 149. For examples of Japanese Buddhist monks and medicines in China, see Sesson Yūbai's 雪村友梅 (1290–1346) poem thanking the Chinese monk Shiqiao 石橋 for providing medicine (*Bingashū,* in *Gozan bungaku zenshū,* vol. 1, pp. 530–531); Chūgan Engetsu's 中巌円月 (1300–1375) riveting poem "In China: Sick with Malarial Fever" (David Pollack, *Zen Poems of the Five Mountains,* p. 141); or Zekkai Chūshin's 絶海中津 (1336–1405) poem written to an acquaintance from his home province in Japan who was ill in Nanjing, and the poem to physician Geng Langzhong 耿郎中, whom he compared to the legendary healers Yu Fu 兪跗 and Bian Que 扁鵲, thanking him for the medicines and treatments that he provided (*Shōkenkō,* in *Gozan bungakushū,* pp. 74–75, no. 35; and *Gozan bungakushū,* p. 51, no. 27).
27. Ritsu is a multifaceted topic. See, for example, Lori Meeks, *Hokkeji and the Reemergence of Female Monasticism in Medieval Japan;* David Quinter, "The

Shingon Ritsu School and the Mañjuśrī Cult in the Kamakura Period"; and Janet Goodwin, *Alms and Vagabonds.*

28. See Abé Ryūchi, "Mantra, Hinin and the Feminine: On the Salvational Strategies of Myōe and Eizon," p. 122.
29. On aspects of healing and medicine in the Ippen Scroll, see Sunagawa Hiroshi, "Ishō toshite no Ippen," and Shinmura Taku, "Yamai no zuzō hyōgen." For reference to the urine, see *Tengu zōshi,* text original at pp. 58–59 (sheet 19), printed transcription at p. 168: The scene in question shows two women holding a bamboo tube against Ippen's groin in order to obtain a supply of his urine.
30. David Quinter, "The Shingon Ritsu School and the Mañjuśrī Cult in the Kamakura Period," p. 311; and note 27 noting the centrality of one passage in the *Mañjuśrī Paranirvāna Sutra* to the Ritsu Precept sect (See Quinter, pp. 303–313, for a complete translation of the sutra):

    The Buddha proclaimed to Bhadrapāla: "If people call to mind this Dharma-Prince Mañjuśrī, if they wish to make offerings and cultivate meritorious deeds, then [Mañjuśrī] will transform himself, turning into an impoverished, solitary, or afflicted sentient being, and appear before the practitioners. When people call Mañjuśrī to mind they should practice compassion."

31. 1267.7.23 Hannyaji Monju Engi, translated in Quinter, "Creating Bodhisattvas: Eison, *Hinin,* and the 'Living Mañjuśrī,'" pp. 459–468, at p. 465. Also in Quinter, "The Shingon Ritsu School and the Mañjuśrī Cult in the Kamakura Period," pp. 343–354, at p. 350.
32. The definitive work on Ninshō is now Matsuo Kenji, *Ninshō.* See also Matsuo Kenji, ed., *Eison, Ninshō,* and Wajima Yoshio, *Eison, Ninshō.* For the main source on Ninshō's life, see the *Shōkō Daitokufu.* For a seated sculpture of him, see *Gokuraku Ritsuji shi, Chōkoku kōgei sekizō kenzōbutsu hen,* frontispiece and pp. 96–100. I would like to express my profound gratitude to Gokurakuji Temple for furnishing me with a copy of the *Gokuraku Ritsuji shi* and to Professor Kondō Shigekazu of the Historiographical Institute of Tokyo University for facilitating the process.
33. See Quinter, "The Shingon Ritsu School and the Mañjuśrī Cult in the Kamakura Period," pp. 72–84, 137–140.
34. *Azuma kagami,* Jōkyū 3 (1221).1.27. Additional items were provided to attending priests, and thirty imprisoned criminals were granted pardons; *Azuma kagami,* Hōji 1 (1247).8.20 and Kenchō 2 (1250).3.16.
35. Kōchō 1 (1261).2.20 Kamakura bakufu tsuikahō (*CHSS,* 1:389, 1: 393). On the buying and selling of people, see Thomas Nelson, "Slavery in Medieval Japan."
36. Kōchō 1 (1261).2.20 Kamakura bakufu tsuikahō (*CHSS,* 1:397).

37. See for example Kenkyū 2 (1191).3.28 Go-Toba-in senshi (*KI,* 1:526) or Kangi 3 (1231).11.3 Go-Horikawa tennō senshi (*KI,* 6:4240). Among the numerous items ranging from clothing, to the taking of animal life, to street and bridge repair, we find provisions directing that the ill and the solitary who have been discarded on the roadside be sent to such hospital facilities as the Hiden'in or the Seyaku'in.
38. This is seen most evidently in other portions of the 1261 New Administrative Regulations, where the conduct of Amidist followers is excoriated:

    Item: Prohibiting the holding of drinking parties and the eating of fish and fowl by priests. Drinking parties and eating to surfeit are contrary to precepts. How can this be pardoned? Not only this. It is also reported that when interacting with lay people and children, meat items are being used as snacks and appetizers. This is absolutely contrary to propriety and is to be permanently prohibited. (Kōchō 1 [1261].2.20 Kamakura bakufu tsuikahō [*CHSS,* 1:377])

    Item: Adherents of the Amidist faith. Those who are firm in their practices are excepted from these prohibitions. It has been widely reported that there are those who invite women and engage in lewd and orgiastic behavior, or else eat fish and fowl and are fond of drinking parties. Ward commissioners are hereby ordered to demolish those dwellings [in which such activities have taken place]. The persons themselves are to be expelled from Kamakura. (Kōchō 1 [1261].2.20 Kamakura bakufu tsuikahō [*CHSS,* 1:386])
39. For a useful introduction, see Mabuchi Kazuo, *Kamakura Daibutsu no chūseishi.*
40. On Tokiyori and Lanxi Daolong, see Martin Collcutt, "Lanxi Daolong (1203–1278) at Kenchōji: Chinese Contributions to the Making of Medieval Japanese Rinzai Zen." For the growth of monastic Zen more generally, see Martin Collcut, *Five Mountains: The Zen Monastic Institution in Medieval Japan.*
41. See Carl Steenstrup, *Hōjō Shigetoki.* For translations of Shigetoki's writings, see pp. 143–157 and 162–197.
42. See Fukushima Kaneharu, *Kanezawa Hōjō shi to Shōmyōji,* pp. 122, 131–132, 180. On Sanetoki, see Seki Yasushi, "Hōjō Sanetoki," and Nagai Susumu, *Kanezawa Hōjō shi no kenkyū,* pp. 84–102. On the Kanazawa Bunko and its history, the definitive study is still Seki Yasushi, *Kanazawa bunko no kenkyū.* On portraits, see Murai Shōsuke, *Nanbokuchō no dōran,* p. 250.
43. For information on Jōshun, I have relied upon Hosokawa Ryōichi, ed., *Kanjin Gakushōki—Saidaiji Eison no jiden,* vol. 1, note 12 at pp. 161–162, and notes 14 and 15 at p. 263. Regarding the *Issaikyō,* see too Kanagawa Kenritsu Kanazawa Bunko, ed., *Karamono to Sōban Issaikyō,* plate 48 and

explanation p. 46. For a listing of the *Issaikyō* known to have been imported, see Ōtsuka Norihiro, "Sōban *Issaikyō* no yu'nyū to juyō."

44. For a discussion of the trip, see Mabuchi Kazuo, *Kamakura Daibutsu no chūseishi,* pp. 84–118. For a very useful discussion of the larger context of the trip, see Yoshida Fumio, "Saidaiji Eison no Kantō gekō."

45. See Yoshida Fumio, "Ninshō no shakai jigyō ni tsuite," p. 411.

46. Surviving documentation on Gokurakuji has been assembled in *Gokuraku Ritsuji shi chūsei kinsei hen.* On the naming of Gokurakuji Temple, see Fukushima Kaneharu, *Kanezawa Hōjō shi to Shōmyōji,* p. 122.

47. Ishii Susumu, "Toshi Kamakura ni okeru 'jigoku' no fūkei," pp. 83–85, 90–95; Fukushima Kaneharu, *Kanezawa Hōjō shi to Shōmyōji,* p. 74. Ninshō articulated his approach in a ten-article vow written in 1272 (see Matsuo, *Ninshō,* pp. 123–127). The vows are as follows:

    1. As far as my strength permits, to make the three jewels [Buddha, Dharma, Clergy] flourish.
    2. To be not negligent in the set activities conducted in the morning, the daytime, and at evening, and to attend and take part in morning and nighttime discussions and assemblies.
    3. When traveling around with my three robes and a bowl, to absolutely carry them by myself.
    4. Insofar as I am not ill, not to ride in a carriage or on a horse.
    5. Not to receive special and separate support from a patron.
    6. To exhibit compassion for the solitary, the impoverished, beggars, the lame, and horses and oxen discarded by the roadside.
    7. To make roads in treacherous places, to build bridges over watercourses, to dig wells where there is no water, and to plant medicinal herbs and trees in mountain and field.
    8. To regard as Good Friends people who resent me or indulge in slander against me, and to use expedient means [方便] to aid them.
    9. To permanently abstain from the use of *tenshin* [点心] [small snacks], and in particular to refrain from any foods remaining on the hands while preparing meals.
    10. As to the benefits arising from carrying out these vows which I shall observe, I will not allow the efficacy to remain in my being for even an instant, but will extend it in its entirety to sentient beings in all the worlds in all the ten directions.

48. See Matsuo Kenji, "Hakata Daijōji to chūsei toshi Hakata." For the dispatching of the trade ship, for which venture Gokurakuji received the active backing of the *bakufu,* the Kanezawa family, and the Nagai family of bureaucrats, see Fukushima Kaneharu, *Kanezawa Hōjō shi to Shōmyōji,* pp. 215–233.

49. Hosokawa Ryōichi, "Ninshō no shōgai," p. 119, has speculated that Ninshō had an unfulfilled desire to visit China. He suggests that in 1298, when Ninshō copied out the *Tōseiden emaki* 東征伝絵巻 (Scroll of the Pacification of the East) depicting the journey to Japan of the blind Chinese priest Ganjin (Ch. Jianzhen) 鑑真, Ninshō was symbolically completing his own journey as a bringer of the Precepts to Japan. For Ninshō's interlinear notation, see *Tōseiden emaki* okugaki, in *Gokuraku Ritsuji shi chūsei kinsei hen,* pp. 45–46.
50. This discussion draws upon Yoshida Fumio, "Ninshō no shakai jigyō ni tsuite," pp. 410–412.
51. See the map of Gokurakuji (*Gokurakuji keidai ezu*) reproduced (among other places) in one of the frontispieces to *Gokuraku Ritsuji shi chūsei kinsei hen,* or in Matsuo Kenji, *Chūsei no toshi to hinin,* p. 83. As Matsuo notes, the current map dates from several centuries later, but recent archaeological study has confirmed its accuracy.
52. This discussion draws on Yoshida Fumio, "Ninshō no shakai jigyō ni tsuite," pp. 413–414. The first source is the *Gokurakuji Jūji Junnin ekō fumi* (referred to by Yoshida as *Ninshō tsuizen fumi*): see *Gokuraku Ritsuji shi chūsei kinsei hen,* pp. 92–98, at p. 95 (also in *KI,* 35:27034). The second source is *Genkō Shakusho,* vol. 13, at pp. 202–203.
53. Ryūichi Abé ("Mantra, Hinin, and the Feminine," pp. 122–123) has argued that the determination of numbers of *rai* sufferers cured by Ninshō seems to have resulted from a misdiagnosis, according to the modern medical standard, by which those suffering from skin disorders other then leprosy were counted as lepers. Abé is not entirely incorrect in noting that the figure may have included people suffering skin disorders other than leprosy. Unfortunately, however, he has made the mistake of anachronistically assuming that the modern use of the term *rai* to connote leprosy (Hansen's disease) can be applied to the same term *rai* that we find in the medieval era. Ninshō and others knew their *rai,* and it is clear that the medieval *rai* covered a broader range of skin afflictions than just Hansen's disease. The misdiagnosis, in other words, is that of Abé, not that of medieval Japanese.
54. Saeki Kōji, "Chinese Trade Ceramics in Medieval Japan," p. 174.
55. Ibid., pp. 165–166.
56. Ibid., p. 167. Sadaaki was a central figure in the importation of Chinese goods. See Kanagawa Kenritsu Kanazawa Bunko, ed., *Cha to Kanezawa Sadaaki;* and Nagai Susumu, *Kanezawa Sadaaki.*
57. Murai Shōsuke, *Nanbokuchō no dōran,* pp. 232–237. For reference to a ship being sent to assist the repair of the Great Buddha, see Gentoku 1 (1329).12.3 Sūken (Kanezawa Sadaaki) shojō (*KI,* 39:30790).
58. For a brief introduction, see Saeki Kōji, "Chinese Trade Ceramics in Medieval Japan." For the Nikaidō trade activity, see Yanagihara Toshiaki,

"Chūsei zenki minami Kyūshū no minato to Sōjin kyoryūchi ni kansuru ichi shiron."

59. See Hyungsub Moon, "The Matsura Pirate-Warriors of Northwestern Kyushu in the Kamakura Age," pp. 373–375. The case is also noted in Seno Seiichirō, "Kamakura jidai ni okeru totōsen no sōnan ni miru tokusō ke bōeki dokusen no ichi keitai," and Murai Shōsuke, *Nanbokuchō no dōran,* pp. 229–232.
60. Shōzen notes Qingzhuo as presiding over a major dedication ceremony at Kenchōji in 1326: *Man'anpō,* chapter 39 (*KS,* p. 1014, XXXIX-82). On Qingzhuo, see, briefly, Heinrich Dumoulin, *Zen Buddhism: A History,* pp. 37–38.
61. Shinmura Taku, *Nihon iryō shakai shi no kenkyū,* p. 331.
62. *Ton'ishō*, chapter 21 (*KS*, p. 371, X-161).
63. Kakehi Masahiro, *Mōko shūrai to tokusei rei,* pp. 328–329. For the document, see undated (1320?) Kanezawa Sadaaki shojō (*KI,* 35:27238).
64. Murai Shōsuke, *Nanbokuchō no dōran,* pp. 251–252.
65. *Man'anpō,* chapter 1 (*KS,* p. 52, I-87): The Song person Daoguang did the clean copy; *Man'anpō,* chapter 3 (*KS,* p. 91, III-74): The Song person Daoguang did the clean copy; *Man'anpō,* chapter 6 (*KS,* p. 166, VI-188): Song person Daoguang did the copying; *Man'anpō* chapter 10 (*KS,* p. 268, X-129): The clean copy was done by a Song person.
66. *Man'anpō,* chapter 16 (*KS* p. 471, XVI-6; *KS* p. 488, XVI-72-73). The reference to Yukifuji is of interest here, since it would appear that he had died prior to the completion of the *Ton'ishō.* Accordingly, if the *Hokiron* went into Yukifuji's library while he was still alive, then it cannot have been written after 1302. Alternately, if the reference to the library was to the collection previously owned by Yukifuji or to a library based upon Yukifuji's collection, then this would not hold. In either case, reference to the library's existence is an important piece of information on the bibliographical world of Kamakura.
67. For some background on these families, see Andrew Goble, "The Kamakura Bakufu and Its Officials"; Koizumi Yoshiaki, "Gokenin Nagai shi ni tsuite"; Hosokawa Shigeo, "Mandokoro shitsuji Nikaidō shi ni tsuite"; and Nagai Susumu, *Kanezawa Hōjō shi no kenkyū,* pp. 185–220.
68. On Sadahide, see Nagai Susumu, "Nagai Sadahide no kenkyū," in Nagai's *Kanezawa Hōjō shi no kenkyū,* pp. 194–220; see also pp. 185–191, 250–252, 255–257, 259–260, 367–370.
69. [Enkyō 1 (1308)?].4.14 Nagai Sadahide shojō (*KI,* 31:23503).
70. Undated Nagai Sadahide shojō (*KI,* 31:23528).
71. [Shōchū 2 (1325)?] Bō shojō (*KI,* 37:29058). Cited in Ishihara Akira, "Kajiwara Shōzen no shōgai to sono chosho," p. 1743.

Chapter 2 Song Medicine: A View from Japan

1. For the *Ishinpō* reference, dealing with a formula for Chebulic Myrobalan Pill 訶梨靭丸, see *Man'anpō,* chapter 25 (*KS,* pp. 706–707, XXV-68-71). For the reference to the *Chōsei ryōyōhō,* see *Man'anpō,* chapter 21 (*KS,* p. 576, XXI-39), which notes that the formula for Six-Ingredient Musk Pill 六物麝香丸 is a secret one found in that work.
2. On the reluctance to share titles, see *Gyokuyō,* Yōwa 2 (1182).8.29 (2.572). For examples of recording access: The Wake family's copy of the *Qianjin fang* notes that Nakakage 仲影 (?–1319) copied it in 1277; his son Hirokage 弘影 (?–1349) read it in 1301; another son, Otonari 音成, read it in 1309; and yet another son, Tsugunari 嗣成 (d. 1355), copied it in 1315 and checked that against the Nakakage's 1277 copy (Kosoto Hiroshi, *Chūgoku igaku koten to Nihon,* pp. 446–447). The Tanba family copied *Huangdi neijing mingtang* 黄帝内経明堂 through four generations in 1213, 1244, 1270, and 1296: Kosoto, *Chūgoku igaku koten to Nihon,* pp. 164–165.
3. For a listing of the works cited in the *Ishinpō,* see Kosoto Hiroshi, "*Ishinpō* in'yō bunkenmei sakuin."
4. The 1293 *Honchō shojaku mokuroku* lists *Ishinpō* along with other Japanese works such as *Daidō ruijū hō, Honzō wamyō,* and *Shōchū hō* 掌中方 (Formulas in Hand).The *Ishinpō* is not listed among the holdings of the Heian era's greatest bibliophile, Fujiwara Michinori, though the catalog of his library (*Tsūken nyūdō zōsho mokuroku* 通憲入道蔵書目録) lists pharmaceutical texts such as the *Honzō wamyō* and the Chinese *Daguan bencao* 大観本草. *Gyokuyō,* Kaō 2 (1170).3.2 (1.89) notes that Tanba Norimoto provided a copy of chapter 28 of the *Ishinpō* to Kujō Kanezane.
5. While the *Daguan bencao* was the primary source, Tomotoshi also drew upon such works as the *Taiping huimin Hejiju fang* (hereafter *Hejiju fang:* Formulas of the Pharmacy Service for Great Peace and for the Benefit of People, 1107–1110), *Puji benshi fang* (Effective Formulas for Universal Relief, c. 1150), *Sanyin fang* 三因方 (Treatise on the Three Categories of Pathogenic Factors of Disease, first printed 1174), the *Shizhai baiyi xuan fang* 是斎百一選方 (Shizhai's 101 Selected Formulas, 1197), and the *Waike jingyao* 外科精要 (Essentials of External Medicine, 1263). See Ishihara Akira, "*Honzō iroha shō* kaidai," pp. 622–628. For the Chinese medical works cited, see Mayanagi Makoto, "*Honzō iroha shō* shoin no igaku bunken."
6. This is based on the titles appearing in Kosoto Hiroshi's series of articles dealing with printed texts produced in the Song, Jin, and Yuan: "Hokusō jidai no iyaku sho," "Nansō jidai no iyaku sho," "Kindai no iyaku sho," and "Gendai no iyakusho."

7. For more extensive treatment, see Kosoto Hiroshi, "Volumes of Knowledge: Observations on Song Period Printed Medical Texts."
8. While long known to have been rearranged in the Northern Song, the recent discovery of a Song printed text in Shanghai has now made it apparent that the editors assembled so much material that the best that can be said about the current extant edition is that it was at least based upon some material that was original to Zhang Zhongjing. See Mayanagi Makoto, "*Jingui yaolüe* no seiritsu to genzon hanpon."
9. Kosoto Hiroshi, "Volumes of Knowledge: Observations on Song-Period Printed Medical Texts," p. 220.
10. Guo Xiumei, Kosoto Hiroshi, and Okada Kenkichi, "*Man'anpō* yin zhongguo yishu guankui," p. 129. For a guide to the titles cited in the *Man'anpō,* see this work and Hattori Toshirō, *Kamakura jidai igakushi no kenkyū,* pp. 148–151.
11. Yet even this has value. A case study of the influence of the classic *Shanghan lun* on the pediatrics section of the *Man'anpō* has pointed out that those indirect citations tell us much of the ongoing winnowing process in Chinese medical writing. See Adachihara Akiko, "*Man'anpō* shōnimon ni mirareru *Shanghan lun* no eikyō," pp. 280–292.
12. For the *Ton'ishō,* see Hattori Toshirō, *Kamakura jidai igakushi no kenkyū,* pp. 122–124; for *the Man'anpō,* see the chart inserted at p. 150.
13 Hattori Toshirō, *Kamakura jidai igakushi no kenkyū,* p. 121.
14. Kosoto Hiroshi, *Chūgoku igaku koten to Nihon,* p. 20; Hattori Toshirō, *Kamakura jidai igakushi no kenkyū,* p. 132.
15. For a study of the works cited in the *Youyou xinshu,* see Liu Shukui, "*Youyou xinshu* yinyong yixue wenxian kao." For the count of *Youyou xinshu* citations, see Guo Xiumei and Kosoto Hiroshi, *Man'anpō in'yō shomei sakuin.* For the determination that few formulas are attributed to it, see Adachihara Akiko, "*Man'anpō* no shōnimon ni tsuite," pp. 353–367.
16. *Man'anpō,* chapter 13 (*KS,* p. 321, XIII-95).
17. *Man'anpō,* chapter 13 (*KS,* p. 312, XIII-58).
18. See the editions of the *Furen daquan liangfang* and the *Waike jingyao* in vol. 3 of the *Wakoku Kanseki isho shūsei* series.
19. It is cited in Sun Yunxian's 孫允賢 *Yifang jicheng* 医方集成 (Collection of Medical Formulas, of 1321).
20. The issue is somewhat complicated by the fact that not infrequently, Shōzen notes "the discourse states" without identifying the source from which the information is drawn. It is also possible that "discourse" is plural rather than singular. But for reference, the *Shengji zonglu, Hejiju fang, Youyou xinshu,* and *Sanyin fang* seem to be the most common sources of information for

those sections. For a general overview, see Hattori Toshirō, *Kamakura jidai igakushi no kenkyū,* pp. 100–118, 141–147.

21. For a broader study of women's medicine, see Charlotte Furth, *A Flourishing Yin: Gender in China's Medical History, 960–1665.* The first work on women's medicine seems to be the Tang-period work of Zan Yin, the *Jingxiao chanbao* 経効産宝 (Tested Treasuries in Obstetrics).
22. For information on this important figure, see Morris Rossabi, *Khubilai Khan: His Life and Times.*
23. In a related area, the reader is directed to a compilation that reflects the cosmopolitan influences that coursed through the Yuan medico-culinary regime. See Paul Buell and Eugene Anderson, *A Soup for the Qan: Chinese Dietary Medicine of the Mongol Era as Seen in Hu Szu-Hui's* Yin-shan cheng-yao.
24. Also referred to as the *Leizheng puji benshi fang* and the *Benshi fang.* Xu subsequently produced a follow-up volume, the *Leizheng puji benshi fang houfang,* containing a further three hundred formulas. Five other of his works have not survived.
25. See Kosoto Hiroshi, "*Taiping huimin Hejiju fang* kaidai," p. 2. For a recent study of the compilation and emendation of the various editions, see Suzuki Tatsuhiko, "*Hejiju fang* no Shōkō, Hōkei, Jun'yū jidai no hensan hōhō to ito," and his "*Hejiju fang* no zōho nendai no mondai."
26. Ishihara Akira, "*Honzō iroha shō* kaidai," p. 627.
27. *Man'anpō,* chapter 13 (*KS,* p. 327, XIII-119–120). The five fragrances are costus, cloves, aloes, frankincense, and *agastache.*
28. *Man'anpō,* chapter 13 (*KS,* p. 309, XIII-48), headnote, refers to both a "separate edition Service Formulas" 別本局方 and to an annotated and expanded *Daquan Hejiju fang* 大全和剤局方 (Great Complete Formulas of the Pharmacy Service).
29. For the first reference, see *Man'anpō,* chapter 49 (*KS,* p. 1295, XLIX-104). For the second, see *Man'anpō,* chapter 46 (*KS,* p. 1186, XLVI-9), and also *Youyou xinshu,* chapter 27, section 11. The *Man'anpō* phrasing is more extensive than that found in either the *Youyou xinshu* or the *Hejiju fang* and includes directions on preparation that are not in the editions of *Youyou xinshu* and *Hejiju fang* that I consulted.
30. *Youyou xinshu,* chapter 40, sections 13–15. *Man'anpō,* chapter 49 (*KS,* pp. 1295–1299, XLIX-101–118).
31. See, for example, a headnote in chapter 13 of *Man'anpō,* where Shōzen quotes Chu Yushi's *Yangsheng biyong fang.* The form of the headnote is the same as for other works such as *Hejiju fang,* which he cites and which we know to have been available to him: *Man'anpō,* chapter 13 (*KS,* p. 304, above XIII-27).
32. *Man'anpō,* chapter 12 (*KS,* p. 293, XII-34).

33. *Man'anpō,* chapter 22 (*KS,* p. 643, XXII-167).
34. *Ton'ishō,* chapter 13 (*KS,* p. 239, VII-73).
35. *Ton'ishō,* chapter 18 (*KS,* p. 329, IX-168).
36. *Ton'ishō,* chapter 35 (*KS,* p. 541, XVI-103-104). See also *Man'anpō,* chapter 40 (*KS,* pp. 1022–1023, XL-31-34).
37. *Man'anpō,* chapter 22 (*KS,* p. 643, XXII-167).
38. *Man'anpō,* chapter 22 (*KS,* p. 648, XXII-185-186; and the headnote at XXII-185). Hattori Toshirō, *Igaku,* p. 78, notes that this comment is to be found in the *Ton'ishō,* but this reference seems mistaken.
39. *Man'anpō,* chapter 23 (*KS,* p. 661–662, XXIII-51-53).
40. *Man'anpō,* chapter 14 (*KS,* pp. 393–394, XIV-146-148). Shōzen has here jumbled the names of two people, the Song priest physician Chu Yushi 初虞世 and the Tang bureaucrat Yu Shinan 虞世南. The latter is listed instead of the former at least six times in the *Man'anpō.* For example, *Man'anpō,* chapter 1 (*KS,* p. 40, I-42) headnote, and the citations in the main body of the text. However, Chu is correctly referred to at least forty times: e.g., *Man'anpō,* chapter 13 (*KS,* p. 304, XIII-27), and *Man'anpō,* chapter 14 (*KS,* p. 391, XIV-138).
41. *Man'anpō,* chapter 52 (*KS,* p. 1446, LII-83).
42. *Ton'ishō,* chapter 36 (*KS,* p. 557–558, XVII-44-45).
43. *Ton'ishō,* chapter 27 (*KS,* p. 422, XIII-10). For a useful elaboration of Sun's point, see Sabine Wilms, "'Ten Times More Difficult to Treat': Female Bodies in Medical Texts from Early Imperial China," especially pp. 88–93.
44. *Man'anpō,* chapter 32 (*KS,* p. 876, XXXII-35).
45. *Man'anpō,* chapter 32 (*KS,* p. 881, XXXII-57, headnote).
46. *Man'anpō,* chapter 32 (*KS,* pp. 884–885, XXXII-70-71).
47. *Man'anpō,* chapter 32 (*KS,* p. 869, XXXII-9-10).
48. *Ton'ishō,* chapter 12 (*KS,* p. 237, VII-67).
49. *Man'anpō,* chapter 32 (*KS,* pp. 875–876, XXXII-34-35). The phrases in the final sentence are taken from two classical Chinese stories. In the first story, which appears in *Hanfeizi* (see Burton Watson, *Han Fei Tzu: Basic Writings,* p. 97), after a hare ran into a tree stump and killed itself, a farmer gave up farming with its predictable yield in favor of waiting for another hare to appear, run into the stump, and thus provide food. The second phrase refers to a story, found in the *Spring and Autumn Annals,* of carving a notch into the side of a boat from which a sword has fallen into the sea and assuming that the mark on the boat will indicate the location of the sword, quite oblivious of the fact that the boat floats around and never keeps to the same position.
50. See, for example, *Tamon'in nikki,* Eiroku 11 (1568).6.9 (2.76), for a method of correcting breech births that involves shaving the woman's head, rubbing

ointment on the shaven spot to draw the child back up, then applying ointment on the sole of the woman's foot to draw the infant back down correctly.

51. *Man'anpō,* chapter 34 (*KS,* p. 903, XXXIV-11).
52. *Man'anpō,* chapter 34 (KS p. 996, XXXIX-12).
53. *Man'anpō,* chapter 34 (*KS,* p. 998, XXXIX-17). See too the immediately preceding discussion on tying the umbilical cord (*KS,* p. 997–998, XXXIX-15~17).
54. *Man'anpō,* chapter 34 (*KS,* p. 914, XXXIV-55~56); for the full passage of Shōzen's remarks, see (*KS,* p. 914–915, XXXIV-55~59).
55. *Man'anpō,* chapter 34 (*KS,* p. 912, XXXIV-47~48).

Chapter 3 A Silk Road of Pharmaceuticals and Formulas

1. *Shaken Nichiroku,* Bunmei 18 (1486).7.15.
2. So much pepper was shipped through Japan that in Korea it was thought to be a Japanese product, which of course it was not: Ts'ao Yung-ho, "Pepper Trade in East Asia," p. 242. An early-fifteenth-century Chinese work, the *Jingzhilu* 敬止録 (Record of Things Esteemed and Halted), which details items from Japan presented as part of the tribute trade to China, likewise lists a number of Southeast Asian items among Japanese tribute goods: See Nakajima Gakushō, "Eiroku nenkan no Nichimin chōkō bōeki," pp. 77–80. On the other hand, Japanese residents in Kyoto were aware that musk and cloves were from Southern Barbarian regions (Nanban) and brought to Japan via Ryukyu: Seki Shūichi, "Kōryō no michi to Nihon, Chōsen," pp. 267–268.
3. The most useful survey of early pharmaceutical history remains Okazaki Kanzō, *Kusuri no rekishi,* particularly pp. 1–92. For a broader treatment of trade and interaction from early times, see Charlotte von Verschuer, *Across the Perilous Sea: Japanese Trade with China and Korea from the Seventh to Seventeenth Centuries,* and Bruce Batten, *Gateway to Japan: Hakata in War and Peace, 500–1300.*
4. Tōno Haruyuki, *Kentōshi to Shōsōin,* pp. 184–185, notes that Hōryūji Temple preserves a box originally containing such aromatics as aloes and white sandalwood. The name of the merchant who had originally supplied them is branded on the box in Pahlavi script (late-Sassanian cursive script).
5. For a discussion of the earliest inventory registry from 756, see Mori Shikazō, "Shōsōin yakubutsu to shuju yakuchō," in Asahina Yasuhiko, ed., *Shōsōin no yakubutsu,* pp. 17–67. See also Okazaki Kanzō, *Kusuri no rekishi,* pp. 45–50. For a table of the depletion of the original stores between 756 and 856, see Mori Shikazō, *Honzōgaku kenkyū,* pp. 152–155. For a 764 request from the Imperial Pharmacy (Seyakuin) requesting further supplies

of cassia since the exhaustion of their stock brought the compounding of medicines to a halt, see Hayakawa Shōhachi, *Shoku Nihongi,* pp. 65–67. For a study of the paper made of recycled documents upon which notations of weight were recorded and that was used to wrap stocks of cinnabar, see Nojiri Tadashi, "Kinryō kisai kara mita Shōsōin tan uramonjo no kenkyū."

6. For further information, see Koizumi Enjun, "Mikkyō to honzō," and Ariga Yōen, *Kō to bukkyō.*
7. For a discussion, see Mori Shikazō, *Honzōgaku kenkyū,* pp. 244–339.
8. See *Shinsarugaku ki,* pp. 150–151. For a translation of all of the items in which the merchant dealt, see Batten, *Gateway to Japan,* table 7, p. 115.
9. *Kōan yonen ikoku onkitō ki,* entry for 1281.4.22 (*ZGR,* p. 178). My reference from Koizumi Enjun, "Bukkyō to mikkyō," p. 47.
10. *Ton'ishō,* chapter 17 (*KS,* p. 314, IX-106-107). The formula consists of three items: the skin of chebula fruit *(Terminalia chebula),* ephedra *(Ephedra sinica),* and Wax Tea. The items to be used in the compounding of the Wax Tea are tea *(Thea),* rind of pomegranate *(Punica granatum),* and beeswax (*ōra* 黄臈, i.e. 黄臘, 黄蠟). For an excellent introduction to Wax Tea, see Iwama Machiko, *Cha no iyakushi,* pp. 217–267. The present reference from the *Ton'ishō* supplements those that Iwama notes from the *Man'anpō* (Iwama, ibid., pp. 139–140).
11. (1323) Hōjō Sadatoki jusannen imi kuyō ki (*Kamakura shishi shiryō hen 2,* Engakuji monjo doc. 69, pp. 76–128, at pp. 76–77).
12. Shibata Shōji ed., *Hōryūji shozō Iyaku chōzai koshō,* pp. 35 and 50. The fifteen other items were rhubarb, ginger, fennel, Chinese sesame, musk, Chinese licorice, betel nut, myrobalic chebulan, cinnabar, Burmese rosewood, aloes, white sandalwood, cloves, croton, and fossil bones.

    The Wake and Tanba seem to have maintained their own hoard of materia medica as a matter of course. One author, writing in the fifteenth century, noted that the Wake and Tanba families had stores of such imported items as ginseng, Borneo camphor, Dragon's Blood, birthwort root, black pepper, wild Siamese cardamom, lesser galangal, cassia, licorice, Sichuan lovage, Chinese angelica, croton, rhubarb, realgar, dried tiger gallbladder, cinnabar, and honey-ball (honeyed bolus): see *Sekiso ōrai,* p. 609.
13. The *Fukudenpō* is generally dated to the 1360s, but it may have been compiled as late as the mid-1400s. See Sasaki Toshikazu, "Hakubutsukan shomoku shikō Teishitsu bon no bu Igakukan hon hen, *Yūrin Fukudenpō* ni tsuite."
14. For a convenient tabulation, see Takahashi Shintarō, "Chūgoku no yakubutsu ryōhō to sono eikyō," pp. 414–415.
15. Ibid., pp. 419, 420.
16. For a picture of the medicine grinder used at Gokurakuji Temple, see Matsuo Kenji, *Ninshō,* p. 150. A number of the other items are depicted in the scene

from the *Fukutomi zōshi* 福富草紙 (Scroll of Fukutomi), pp. 61–62, where Fukutomi's wife is obtaining medicine to treat his acute diarrhea caused by the ingestion of ten morning glory seeds. For a translation of the story, which revolves around his effort to become a master entertainer specializing in flatulent arias, see Virginia Skord, *Tales of Tears and Laughter.* For a more detailed study, see James Ulak, "Fukutomi Zōshi: The Genesis and Transmutation of a Medieval Japanese Scatalogical Tale."

17. See *Fukudenpō,* vol. 11 (*KS,* pp. 929–935), dealing with measurements; Takahashi Shintarō, "Chūgoku no yakubutsu ryōhō to sono eikyō," pp. 419–421. Understanding these measurements still exercises scholars: see Watanabe Takeshi, Komai Hiroyuki, and Nakajima Kōji, "Ganjin ōshō no hihō Kariroku gan no saiken to *Ishinpō* fūbyō hen, gendaiyaku no goyaku."
18. *Chōsei ryōyōhō,* chapter 15, "Yaku kin ryō shō gō hō," pp. 173–174. Renki informs the reader that according to the *Classic,* whereas there used to be only [for weight] *shu* 銖 and *ryō* 両, now there were ten *sho* 黍 for one *shu* 銖, six *shu* to one *bu* 分, four *bu* to a *ryō,* and sixteen *ryō* to a *kin* 斤. On the volume of a *shō,* Renki notes the difference between small and large medicinal *shō,* what constitutes a *shō* for decoction 湯 and for powder 散 medicines, and what systems are in use in the *Yakuden* 薬殿 (Medicine Hall) and the *Ten'yakuryō* 典薬寮 (Bureau of Medicine) respectively.
19. *Man'anpō,* chapter 13 (*KS,* p. 329, XIII-125–126). For other examples of making this point that ten *sen* make one *ryō,* see *Man'anpō,* chapter 13 (*KS,* p. 339, XIII-168), or *Man'anpō,* chapter 51 (*KS,* p. 1341, LI-92). On this latter occasion, he notes that "there are four *ryō* of fresh ginger. Ten *sen* make one *ryō,* thus forty *sen* weighs at four *ryō;* and with the jujubes at forty-nine *kin,* since Japanese jujubes are smaller it will be 100–200 *kin.*"
20. *Man'anpō,* chapter 15 (*KS,* p. 449, XV-134–135).
21. *Man'anpō,* chapter 31 (*KS,* p. 865, XXXI-115–117). We have no further information about this work. For another example of Shōzen, dealing with a formula from *Huorenshu,* see *Man'anpō,* chapter 42 (*KS,* p. 1081, XLII-56–57): "I say that four *shō* are four large *sakazuki,* a half *shō* is half a *sakazuki;* the introduction to the *Bencao* states that 'in sum one *shō* is patterned on one large *sakazuki,* five *gō* are patterned on a medium *sakazuki,* and three *gō* are patterned on one small *sakazuki.*'"
22. *Man'anpō,* chapter 36 (*KS,* p. 933, XXXVI-7).
23. *Man'anpō,* chapter 15 (*KS,* p. 449, XV-134–135).
24. *Man'anpō,* chapter 10 (*KS,* p. 262, X-103); *Man'anpō,* chapter 11 (*KS,* p. 278, XI-36).
25. *Man'anpō,* chapter 15 (*KS,* p. 444, XV-116). Shōzen also adjusted doses for moxibustion treatment. He notes that whereas the dosage for one moxa

treatment was listed as five cones, depending upon the size and age of the infant or child, five to ten or twenty to thirty cones were to be applied: *Man'anpō,* chapter 49 (*KS,* p. 1063, XLI-89).

26. In his *Idanshō* (Conversations on Medicine), Tomotoshi notes such things as that people didn't realize that the sweet trout 鮎 referred to in lists of permitted and prohibited foods for sick people in fact indicated catfish 鯰 or that Japanese raccoon dog 狸 in fact indicated cat 猫, and that he himself failed to recognize a variant name for root of pokeberry. See *Idanshō,* section titled "The Necessity of Sorting Out Names of Medicines" (*yakumei bunbetsu subeki koto*): Minobe Shigekatsu, *Idanshō,* p. 159.
27. See chapters 47 and 48 of the *Ton'ishō.* These appear to be the precursor for the essay *Shōmi kagami* in the *Man'anpō.*
28. Ishihara Akira, "Kajiwara Shōzen no shōgai to sono chosho," p. 1737.
29. *Man'anpō,* chapter 59 (*KS,* p. 1626, LIX-144).
30. See, for example, *Man'anpō,* chapter 62 (*KS,* p. 1725, LXII-111~112).
31. *Man'anpō,* chapter 17 (*KS,* p. 511, XVII-91~92).
32. *Man'anpō,* chapter 3 (*KS,* p. 78, III-23); *Man'anpō,* chapter 49 (*KS,* p. 1284, XLIX-60); *Man'anpō,* chapter 49 (*KS,* p. 1285, XLIX-62).
33. *Man'anpō,* chapter 45 (*KS,* p. 1183, XLV-125).
34. *Man'anpō,* chapter 40 (*KS,* p. 1037, XL-92).
35. *Man'anpō,* chapter 61 (*KS,* p. 1669, LXI-13); *Man'anpō,* chapter 61 (*KS,* p. 1689, LXI-94); *Man'anpō,* chapter 61 (*KS,* p. 1694, LXI-114); *Man'anpō,* chapter 61 (*KS,* p. 1695, LXI-119); *Man'anpō,* chapter 62 (*KS,* p. 1700, LXII-14); *Man'anpō,* chapter 62 (*KS,* p. 1705, LXII-34); *Man'anpō,* chapter 61 (*KS,* p. 1693, LXI-112).
36. *Man'anpō,* chapter 62 (*KS,* p. 1716, LXII-73); *Man'anpō,* chapter 3 (*KS,* p. 90, III-69).
37. *Man'anpō,* chapter 59 (*KS,* p. 1625, LIX-139); *Man'anpō,* chapter 59 (*KS,* p. 1624, LIX-136); *Man'anpō,* chapter 61 (*KS,* p. 1689, LXI-95); *Man'anpō,* chapter 61 (*KS,* p. 1693, LXI-109).
38. *Ton'ishō,* chapter 24 (*KS,* pp. 407–408, XII-59~62).
39. *Man'anpō,* chapter 52 (*KS,* p. 1406, LII-168).
40. See respectively *Man'anpō,* chapter 31 (*KS,* p. 851, XXXI-62), "Large jujubes twelve granules, Japanese jujubes are small so use thirty-four"; *Man'anpō,* chapter 53 (*KS,* p. 1444, LIII-78), "Use twelve large dried jujubes, if Japanese jujubes does one use fifty?"; *Man'anpō,* chapter 52 (*KS,* p. 1409, LII-179), "I say that the Japanese jujube is smaller."
41. *Ton'ishō,* chapter 35 (*KS,* pp. 536–537, XVI-82~85).
42. *Man'anpō,* chapter 52 (*KS,* p. 1406, LII-168).
43. *Idanshō,* Minobe, p. 159. Tomotoshi was unsure of the difference between Japanese mandarin peel 橘皮 *(Citrus reticulata)* and tangerine peel 陳皮

(also *Citrus reticulata*) but felt one should use the tangerine peel brought into Japan by the Chinese.

44. *Man'anpō,* chapter 21 (*KS,* p. 580, XXI-54-55).
45. *Man'anpō,* chapter 41 (*KS,* p. 1049, XLI-35).
46. *Man'anpō,* chapter 43 (*KS,* pp. 1115, 1116, XLIII-90-91). Shōzen notes that "As to the recipe for Silver Liquid Pill 銀液丹 found in volume nineteen of the *Youyou xinshu,* as well as the Cinnabar Pill 朱砂圓 [noted in the] *Wanquan fang* 万全方 (Myriad Complete Formulas), all the ingredients are difficult to obtain, so I haven't quoted them here. Such formulas as Purple Prime Pill 紫元子, Storax Pill 蘇合香圓, and Trembling Powder 惶々散 are also good."
47. A Chinese work of 1387 notes its existence in Japan (Maejima Norimoto, "Nihon kodai no kōhaku no michi"), and it is listed in a fifteenth-century register of tribute items presented to the Ming court (Nakajima Gakushō, "Eiraku nenkan no Nichimin chōgu bōeki," pp. 77–78). It may have been a transshipped item, like pepper.
48. See, respectively, *Man'anpō,* chapter 21 (*KS,* p. 600, XXI-135); *Man'anpō,* chapter 15 (*KS,* p. 443, XV-111-112); *Man'anpō,* chapter 49 (*KS,* p. 1293, XLIX-94).
49. See *Man'anpō,* chapter 21 (*KS,* p. 600, XXI-135), headnote.
50. *Man'anpō,* chapter 38 (*KS,* p. 984, XXXVIII-32-33). Here Shōzen remarks that the original source *[Furen] Daquan liangfang* had also noted that they were hard to get.
51. *Man'anpō,* chapter 3 (*KS,* p. 78, III-23). This formula appears to be taken from *Shengji zonglu;* see *Shengji zonglu,* chapter 11 (vol. 1, pp. 325–326).
52. *Man'anpō,* chapter 36 (*KS,* p. 934, XXXVI-11).
53. I have benefited greatly from the detailed studies of Adachihara Akiko, "*Manan'pō* shōnimon ni mirareru *Shanghan lun* no eikyō" and "*Man'anpō* no shōnimon ni tsuite."
54. The information here is primarily drawn from Adachihara Akiko, "*Man'anpō* shōnimon ni mirareru *Shanghan lun* no eikyō," pp. 282–287.
55. Nakamura Teruko, Kawaguchi Naomi, and Endō Jirō, "*Hejiju fang* shōkan hen no kentō."
56. Nakamura Teruko, Matsuzaki Aiko, and Endō Jirō, "*Hejiju fang* ni okeru hōkōsei ken'i yaku no kentō – seiiki no igaku no eikyō ni tsuite"; Nakamura Teruko, Matsuzaki Aiko, and Endō Jirō, "*Hejiju fang issaiki* hen no kentō"; Nakamura Teruko, Miyamoto Hirokazu, and Endō Jirō, "*Hejiju fang* ni mirareru seizai no tokuchō."
57. There were also changes in the usage of Chinese materia medica. From the *Waitai miyao fang* to the *Hejiju fang,* one can note a substantial increase in the use of spicebush, Dahurian angelica, perilla, immature orange peel, and

Chinese atractylodes; about the same use of ginger and cinnamon bark; and a drop in the use of magnolia, big-head atractylodes, wild ginger, and Chinese angelica.

58. The following is based on Nakamura Teruko, Matsuzaki Aiko, and Endō Jirō, "*Hejiju fang* ni okeru hōkōsei ken'i yaku no kentō," table 5, p. 156.

59. Birthwort root was, however, one of the four Western-origin drugs listed in the *Waitai miyao.*

60. Note, for example, that the privately printed *Weishi jiacang fang* of 1227, which represented current local clinical knowledge and which was used by Shōzen, has a chapter devoted to ailments of the "all forms of [disorders of] qi". Chapter 2 of the *Weishi jiacang fang* lists such Western-origin items as costus root, black pepper, fennel, asafoetida, long pepper, lesser galangal, dry ginger, *zedoary,* spikenard, cardamom, nutmeg, clove, and sandalwood. Chapter 1 also lists Western-origin items such as such as frankincense, myrrh, *agastache*, and Dragon's Blood.

61. For more detailed treatment of this topic, see Andrew Edmund Goble, "Images of Illness: Interpreting the Medieval *Scrolls of Affliction.*"

62. *Gotai miwakeshū,* chapter 13, 51-A. See also Hattori Toshirō, *Muromachi jidai igakushi no kenkyū,* p. 233.

63. See Sonja Arntzen, *Ikkyū and the Crazy Cloud Anthology,* pp. 175–177, citing the prose introduction to *Kyōunshū* no. 839: "When Ikkyū was old he contracted the illness of diarrhea. He would recover and then contract it again, two or three times in succession. Everyone said, 'It is dangerous.' But when affairs went against his heart, his vital vapors would escape. Yesterday, as chance would have it, he lost about a hundred sticks of ink that he had been saving. He searched but could not find them. As a result, his spirit was not happy, and the diarrhea threatened to start again. All the attendants turned pale."

64. The comments in *Ton'ishō,* chapter 10 (*KS,* p. 192, VI-10~12) may be paraphrased as follows. Shōzen begins by noting that the hundred illnesses arise from the qi. He then goes on to describe nine qi and how they are affected by different conditions and then notes that texts don't necessarily agree what the nine are. He then notes that there are also said to be seven qi. Following this, he notes that the *Sanyin fang* describes seven emotions and lists the ways in which those emotions assault different organs of the body. He feels that while nine qi and seven qi are different, they are by and large not all that different and indeed that there are some other varieties that are not listed here. Thus, despite some differences in details, for Shōzen the essential point—that illnesses arise from the workings of qi and emotions—is not in dispute.

65. For the relevant section, see *Ton'ishō,* chapter 12 (*KS,* pp. 222–224, VII-8~13).

66. The story is mentioned in Nathan Sivin, "Emotional Counter-Therapy," p. 12.
67. *Man'anpō,* chapter 13 (*KS,* pp. 331–332, XIII-135~137). His comment that the hundred ailments arise from the qi is found earlier in the chapter also: *Man'anpō,* chapter 13 (*KS,* p. 299, XIII-6).
68. Initial reference from Shinmura Taku, *Nihon iryō shakai shi no kenkyū,* p. 132, n. 7, noting the *Muchū mondō shū* of Musō Kokushi (1275–1351). See *Muchū mondō shū,* "Yūryoku no danna no kitō, tsuketari Tōjin'i Chikō [Zhiguang]," pp. 59–60.
69. *Ton'ishō,* chapter 9 (*KS,* p. 181, V-87~88); *Ton'ishō,* chapter 10 (*KS,* p. 193, VI-14~16); *Man'anpō,* chapter 10 (*KS,* pp. 261–262, X-102~103); *Man'anpō,* chapter 13 (*KS,* p. 302, XIII-17); *Man'anpō,* chapter 15 (*KS,* pp. 448–449, XV-131~135). As to some of the minor differences, two of the materia medica are not common to all the versions; in one case, four versions use aloes while one other uses gypsum; three use costus while two use birthwort root; in two cases, different terms are used for the same item; and one specifies that the rhinoceros horn is to be black.
70. *Man'anpō,* chapter 14 (*KS,* p. 389, XIV-129).
71. *Man'anpō,* chapter 10 (*KS,* pp. 261–262, X-102~103).
72. *Man'anpō,* chapter 14 (*KS,* p. 396, XIV-156).
73. *Ton'ishō,* chapter 10 (*KS,* p. 193, VI-14~16).
74. Adachihara Akiko, "*Man'anpō* no shōnimon ni tsuite," p. 355, notes that there is an example of Shōzen developing a one-ingredient external-use medicine mentioned in the pediatrics section of the *Man'anpō.* Unfortunately, I have yet to locate this.
75. *Man'anpō,* chapter 13 (*KS,* p. 302, XIII-17).
76. It is perhaps no coincidence that the formulas in a fragmentary late-twelfth-century formula manual all deal with acute diarrhea. See Kosoto Hiroshi, "Koisho dankan *Shinpukuji shōzō reihon kanzō-gan tō hō* kō."
77. The Sanskrit term *agada* means free of diseases and as a medicine denotes one that quickly cures all illnesses. The term "*agada* medicine" is also translated in East Asian texts as "no illness medicine" 無病薬 or "not dying medicine" 不死薬 (which will facilitate immortality).
78. *Ton'ishō,* chapter 7 (*KS,* p. 159, IV-191, 192). Seven of the ingredients were of Chinese origin: achyranthes, Baikal skullcap, golden thread, ginseng, madder, big-head atractylodes, and Amur cork tree. Eight were of Western origin: white sandalwood, Burmese rosewood, safflower, turmeric, black pepper, nutgrass, musk, and Sumatra benzoin. In the *Man'anpō,* Shōzen also notes a nutmeg formula for diarrhea that is an oral tradition: *Man'anpō,* chapter 19 (*KS,* p. 525–526, XIX-32~33).

79. *Ton'ishō,* chapter 8 (*KS,* p. 176, V-67). The ingredients were nutmeg, poppy capsules, ginger, and the Chinese-origin Chinese licorice.
80. I have not encountered any 禾嘉散. However, a 嘉禾散 (as well as the Stomach Calming Powder noted here) is included in the "all forms of disorder of qi" sections of the *Hejiju fang* and in *Man'anpō,* chapter 13 (*KS,* p. 304, XIII-27-28). 嘉禾散 is also noted, with virtually identical ingredients, in another work used by Shōzen, the 1283 *Lingnan weisheng fang* 嶺南衛生方 (Formulas for Safeguarding Life in Lingnan), pp. 72–73.
81. *Man'anpō,* chapter 19 (*KS,* p. 525, XIX-31-32).

Chapter 4 Leprosy, Buddhist Karmic Illness, and Song Medicine

1. For a useful overview of *rai* in medieval Japan, see Kanai Kiyomitsu, *Chūsei no raija to sabetsu.* See also Fujino Yutaka, ed., *Rekishi no naka no "raija";* Kuroda Hideo, "Chūsei minshū no hifu kankaku to kyōfu," in *Kyōkai no chūsei, shōchō no chūsei,* pp. 233–258; Yokota Noriko, "*Monoyoshi* kō: Kinsei Kyoto no raija ni tsuite"; and Suzuki Noriko, "Shodai Manase Dōsan no rai igaku." For the idea of multiple cultural meanings, I am drawing on William Johnston's depiction of tuberculosis in modern times: see *The Modern Epidemic: A History of Tuberculosis in Japan,* p. 155.
2. See the photographs, illustration, and discussion in Hirata Kazuaki, "Kamakura shutsudo jinkotsu no kotsubyōhen: Yuigahama minami iseki shutsudo jinkotsu o chūshin ni," pp. 30–31.
3. For some discussion of this, see Andrew Edmund Goble, "Images of Illness: Interpreting the Medieval *Scrolls of Afflictions.*"
4. For the first, see *Iyaku chōzai koshō* (An Old Work on Compounding Medicines), [51] at pp. 36, 51; for the second, see *Gotai miwakeshū* (Collection on the Five Portions of the Body), chapter 17, 85-B.
5. The youngest child of the leading court aristocrat, Saionji Kintsune 西園寺公経 (1171–1244), was so ashamed of contracting white *rai* that he entered and died in seclusion: *Minkeiki* Bun'ei 4 (1267).2.7 (9:257). A thirteenth-century anecdote reveals that the mere suspicion that a chief priest of a shrine had contracted *rai* would be grounds for his removal and prompted him to seek medical advice as to whether he had contracted the affliction: *Kokon chomonjū* (*NKBT,* pp. 240–241; *KT,* pp. 164–165). The *NKBT* text notes that the affliction was determined to be not *rai* but *hakudan* "white sores," a type of ringworm. The *KT* text notes that the affliction was "white *rai.*" These versions provide two different diagnoses, with different social implications for each. In any event, the point is the concern exhibited by a person who thought that he had contracted *rai.*

6. Kamakura era oaths regularly note white *rai* and black *rai* among the punishments for breaking oaths. See Kuroda Hideo, *Kyōkai no chūsei, shōchō no chūsei,* pp. 233–258. For a sense of the viciousness with which those thought to have contracted *rai* could be described, we have the following gleeful description from the famous priest Ikkyū (1394–1481) regarding the death of a hated rival: "He became ill, but it was not an ordinary illness. Little by little his hair and eyebrows fell out, and from the sixth day of the fifth moon, his body began rotting from the hips down. Later pus oozed out from his throat and blood poured forth so that from the sixth moon he was continually vomiting. His disciples did not recognize leprosy, but when the priests inside the temple and their servants began talking with people outside, some said 'This is leprosy.' On the twenty-seventh day of the sixth moon, he died and his disciples burned his body to the rear of Daiyu-an (a Daitokuji subtemple). Such was against the law since this was an imperial temple." Jon Covell, *Unravelling Zen's Red Thread,* pp. 140–141. For a story of visiting leprosy upon a person who is disliked, see Susan Matisoff, "Holy Horrors," p. 252.
7. See, for example, Bun'ei 1 (1264).12.13 Nichiren shojō (*KI,* 12:9194; translated in the Gosho Translation Committee, ed., *The Writings of Nichiren Daishōnin,* [hereafter *WND*] no. 10, "Encouragement to a Sick Person"); [Bun'ei 12 (1275).2?] Nichiren shojō (*KI,* 15:11810; *WND,* no. 129, "On Prolonging One's Lifespan"); [Kenji 1 (1275)].11.3 Nichiren shojō (*KI,* 16:12102; *WND,* no. 76, "On Curing Karmic Disease"); Kōan 1 (1278).6.26 Nichiren shojō (*KI,* 17:13095; *WND,* no. 120, "The Two Kinds of Illness").
8. Koremune Tomotoshi, in his *Idanshō.* See Minobe Shigekatsu, ed., *Idanshō,* pp. 190–192.
9. In the fourteenth-century *Gotai miwakeshū,* we come across references to a wind-warm disease that is not *raibyō* and to the appearance of snake sores on feet, hands, or nose that are itchy and cannot be treated with moxibustion, indicating that *rai* has been contracted. *Gotai miwakeshū,* chapter 3, 13-A; chapter 12, 48-A. The parts that constituted the body were variously defined, but any combination was intended to refer to the entire body. An early cataloging referred to skin and hair, veins, flesh, sinew, and bone. Later definitions incorporated among the five such things as the head, two arms, two legs, neck, chest, torso, and so on.
10. See Hattori Toshirō, *Kamakura jidai igakushi no kenkyū,* pp. 110–111, 129–133; Kanai Kiyomitsu, *Chūsei no raija to sabetsu,* pp. 31–35. Some scholars have selectively taken Shōzen's comments as reflecting a Buddhist standpoint that provided ideological justification for discrimination against *rai* sufferers, though others suggest that his information was unable to overcome entrenched prejudice in favor of the view of *rai* as a karmic illness.

See, for example, Kobayashi Shigefumi, "Kodai chūsei raija to shūkyō: Sabetsu to kyūzai," p. 17; Kanai Kiyomitsu, *Chūsei no raija to sabetsu,* p. 35. As I hope to show, however, these views all require reevaluation.

11. I am following the transcription in the *KS* edition of the *Ton'ishō.* The unpaginated Naikaku Bunko text refers to "wind evil worms."
12. *Ton'ishō,* chapter 34 (*KS,* pp. 518–519, XVI-12~14).
13. *Ton'ishō,* chapter 34 (*KS,* p. 527, XVI-47~48).
14. Separate from medicinal baths, hot baths were prescribed to help patients who had contracted other problems. For example, Shōzen notes that when *kasahoroshi* (a fever-related rash associated with colds) was contracted, a Chinese bath 唐風呂 must be used: *Ton'ishō,* chapter 34 (*KS,* p. 528, XVI-50).
15. *Ton'ishō,* chapter 34 (*KS,* p 532, XVI-65).
16. *Ton'ishō,* chapter 34 (*KS,* p. 521, XVI-24).
17. *Ton'ishō,* chapter 34 (*KS,* p. 517–518, XVI-7~11).
18. *Ton'ishō,* chapter 34 (*KS,* p. 529, XVI-54~55).
19. *Man'anpō,* chapter 52 (*KS,* p. 1397–1398, LII-130~135).
20. *Ton'ishō,* chapter 34 (*KS,* pp. 528, XVI-49).
21. *Ton'ishō,* chapter 40 (*KS,* p. 605, XIX-42~43).
22. *Ton'ishō,* chapter 34 (*KS,* p. 526–527, XVI-42~45).
23. *Ton'ishō,* chapter 34 (*KS,* p. 526, XVI-42).
24. *Ton'ishō,* chapter 34 (*KS,* p. 530, XVI-63).
25. *Ton'ishō,* chapter 40 (*KS,* p. 605, XIX-43).
26. *Ton'ishō,* chapter 34 (*KS,* p. 526, XVI-42).
27. *Ton'ishō,* chapter 34 (*KS,* p. 526, XVI-44).
28. *Ton'ishō,* chapter 34 (*KS,* p. 530, XVI-62).
29. Nichiren, for example, notes such figures as Shennong, Huangdi, Hua Tuo, Vimalakirti, and skilled physicians such as Water Holder, Water Carrier, Jivaka, and Bian Que. See [Kenji 1 (1275)].11.3 Nichiren shojō (*KI,* 16:12102); *WND* No. 76, "On Curing Karmic Disease"; and [Kōan 1 (1278)].6.26 Nichiren shojō (*KI,* 17:13094); *WND* no. 166, "The Treatment of Illness."
30. See *Ton'ishō,* chapter 50 (*KS,* pp. 747–748, XXV-24~25), where Shōzen notes a mantra to be voiced when administering medicines:

> "Praise to the Eastern Region Physician Lapus Lazuli Buddha, the Elevated Jivaka King of Medicine, and the Snowy Mountain Infant (Vimalakirti?)." Facing the east, chant this one time and then after that administer the medicine. The one administering the medicine must have correct and deep intention and must not say the *nenbutsu* while entertaining any doubts. [Otherwise] placing medicine in the mouth and eliminating the painful ailment is just like [putting] cold

water and snow into boiling water. If the chanting is not done as indicated, then the disease will not be cured quickly.

31. "On the next day on an empty stomach, after administering one saucer of plantain, while observing a Healing Buddha mantra and maintaining a mudra, one prays for the assistance of the Wondrous Buddhas 神明佛陀; then daub the changed body with Transcendent's Treasure Medicine 仙宝薬." *Ton'ishō,* chapter 34 (*KS,* p. 525, XVI-39~40).
32. *Ton'ishō,* chapter 34 (*KS,* p. 522, XVI-25~26).
33. *Ton'ishō,* chapter 34 (*KS,* pp. 519–520, XVI-14~17).
34. The *KS* edition lists this as Thousand Skin 千皮, which is perhaps a transcription error caused by the similarity of the characters.
35. *Ton'ishō,* chapter 34 (*KS,* pp. 528–529, XVI-51~53).
36. Karma is a big topic. For a useful introduction, see P. A. Payutto, *Good, Evil and Beyond: Karma in the Buddha's Teachings.*
37. As we see, for example, from comments of the Pure Land figure Rennyo (1415–1499): "Recently, people have been dying in great numbers, reportedly from an epidemic. It is not that they die primarily from the epidemic. It is [because of] determinate [immutable] karma that has been settled from the first moment of our birth. We should not be so deeply surprised by this. And yet when people die at this time, everyone thinks it strange" (*Rennyo shōnin ofumi, T.* 83, no. 2668, p. 800 register c; and Minor and Ann Rogers, *Rennyo: The Second Founder of Shin Buddhism, with a Translation of His Letters,* p. 234, IV-9, "On an Epidemic").

    "Fall and spring have slipped away, and it is already the middle of early summer in this seventh year of Meiō (1498); I have grown old—I am eighty-four. This particular year, however, I have been seriously beset by illness and, as a result, my whole body has suffered—ears, hands, eyes, and feet; I realize, then, that this is in itself the utmost stage of karmic illness, and also the harbinger of birth in the land of utmost bliss." See *Rennyo shōnin ofumi, T.* 83, no. 2668, p. 801, register c; and Minor and Ann Rogers, *Rennyo,* p. 237, IV-13, "Reflections in Early Summer." What I translate as "the utmost stage of karmic illness" *(gōbyō no itari nari)* is rendered by the Rogers as "the outcome of past karma."
38. See *Maka shikan,* chapter 8, *T.* 46, no. 1911, pp. 106–108; Sekiguchi Shindai, *Maka shikan: Zen no shisō genri,* vol. 2, pp. 186–191.
39. For further exploration of Nichiren's engagement of issues of karma and illness and his role as a counselor and healer of the mind, see Andrew Edmund Goble, "Nichiren Calming Karma: Fear, Sickness and Lotus unto Death."
40. [Kenji 1 (1275)].11.3 Nichiren shojō (*KI,* 16:12102); *WND* no. 76, "On Curing Karmic Disease." What I have rendered as "evil spirits" is noted as "devils" in *WND.*

41. [Kōan 1 (1278)].6.26 Nichiren shōjō (*KI,* 17:13094); *WND* no. 166, "The Treatment of Illness." Another shorter letter written on the same day and apparently an accompaniment to the present one makes some identical points and shares some phrasing, so it will not be considered separately here: see Kōan 1 (1278).6.26 Nichiren shojō (*KI,* 17:13095); *WND* no. 120, "The Two Kinds of Illness."
42. *Ton'ishō,* chapter 34 (*KS,* pp. 533, XVI-71-72).
43. *Mahāparinirvāna Sutra,* chapter 22, "On Pure Actions -2," online at http://www.nirvanasutra.org.uk/nirvanasutrap.html.
44. *Mahāparinirvāna Sutra,* chapter 30, "Bodhisattva Highly Virtuous King (D)," online at http://www.nirvanasutra.org.uk/nirvanasutraw.htm.
45. *The Lotus Sutra,* chapter 3, "Simile and Parable." See Burton Watson, trans., *The Lotus Sutra,* pp. 75–77. For a brief look at the issue of illness in the *Lotus Sutra,* see Sasaki Kaoru, *Nichiren to sono shisō,* pp. 379–398.
46. See William LaFleur, "Hungry Ghosts and Hungry People: Somaticity and Rationality in Medieval Japan."
47. Gokurakuji letter, article 50 (*Gokurakuji dono onshōsoku,* pp. 335–336; Carl Steenstrup, *Hōjō Shigetoki,* p. 180).
48. Gokurakuji letter, article 57 (*Gokurakuji dono onshōsoku,* pp. 336–337; Carl Steenstrup, *Hōjō Shigetoki,* p. 183).
49. Gokurakuji letter, article 24 (*Gokurakuji dono onshōsoku,* at p. 328; Carl Steenstrup, *Hōjō Shigetoki,* p. 170).
50. Here I note two letters written by Nichiren. The first is [Bun'ei 12 (1275).2?] Nichiren shojō (*KI,* 15:11810); *WND* no. 129, "On Prolonging One's Life Span," dated by the editors to 1279. In this letter, Nichiren notes that illnesses are of two types, minor and serious, which can be cured by a skilled physician. He also notes that there are two types of karma, immutable and mutable, but that both may be eradicated (thus eradicating the illness for which they might be the cause) by sincere repentance and by belief in the *Lotus Sutra.* In this letter, there is reference to the Indian king Ajātaśatru, and Nichiren notes that Ajātaśatru's boils, which had resisted the ministrations of the physician Jīvaka, were finally cured by the *Lotus Sutra.* To reinforce that example, Nichiren notes that his own mother's illness was cured and her life extended for four years as a result of Nichiren's prayers for her. However, Nichiren also recommends that the woman visit the physician who had treated her earlier and who was concerned about the likely progress of her illness.

    The second letter is the [Kenji 2 (1276)].3.27 Nichiren shojō (*KI,* 16:12270); *WND* no. 82, "The Bow and the Arrow." Nichiren notes,

    > My greatest concern now is your illness. Fully convinced that you should recover your health, you should continue moxibustion

treatment for three years, as regularly as if you had just began. Even those who are free from illness cannot escape the transience of life, but you are not yet old, and because you are a votary of the *Lotus Sutra,* you will not meet an untimely death [i.e., one not determined by karma 非業ノ死]. Your illness surely is not due to karma, but even if it were, you could rely on the power of the *Lotus Sutra* to cure it. . . . Be deeply convinced, then, that your illness cannot possibly persist, and that your life cannot fail to be extended! Take care of yourself, and do not burden your mind with grief.

51. See Kōan 1 (1278).6.26 Nichiren shojō (*KI,* 17:13095); *WND* no. 120, "The Two Kinds of Illness."
52. *Gotai miwakeshū,* chapter 12, 47-B; chapter 15, 68-B.
53. *Ton'ishō,* chapter 18 (*KS,* p. 329, IX-168). Shōzen notes in passing that the ingredients listed in the newly arrived work are slightly different from those for the same medicine, Ox Gallstone Pure Heart Pill 牛黄清心円, that is listed in the *Hejiju fang.*
54. It is included as one of the essays in Kōshū's *Keiran shūyōshū,* chapter 80, at pp. 765–768. Corpse transmitted diseases are generally associated with pulmonary afflictions, but it is not certain with which modern afflictions they might be equated. Sakai Shizu, *Nihon no iryōshi,* p. 145ff., suggests that they might have included such things as insomnia, lethargy-type encephalitis, diabetes, pulmonary tuberculosis, scurvy, and possibly cardiac asthma.
55. *Denshibyō nijūgo hō.* See also Tanaka Fumihide, "Chūsei kenmitsu ji'in ni okeru shūhō no ichi kōsatsu."
56. *Ton'ishō,* chapter 21 (*KS,* pp. 367–368, X-148~149); *Man'anpō,* chapter 26 (*KS,* pp. 731 ff., XXVI-5 ff.). Intestinal colic was caused by exhaustion and coldness of the kidneys as a result of sexual intercourse; colic of the qi was caused by deeply felt emotions such as melancholy, anxiety, fear, and anger that weakened the qi of the kidneys and caused swelling of the scrotum; water colic was so named because lots of fluid emerged if the swelling was lanced; and egg colic was so named because the scrotum was so swollen that it resembled [chicken] eggs.
57. *Sanyin fang,* chapter 14 (pp. 195–196).
58. *Ton'ishō,* chapter 21 (*KS,* p. 368, X-149).
59. *Man'anpō,* chapter 26 (*KS,* p. 734, XXVI-16~17).
60. See *Ton'ishō,* chapter 9 (*KS,* pp. 179–180, V-78~83). For the comment about washing away in a river, see *Ton'ishō,* chapter 9 (*KS,* p. 184, V-100).
61. For the full citation from chapter 4 of the *Rencun Sunshi zhibing huofa mifang,* see *Man'anpō,* chapter 15 (*KS,* pp. 457–468, XV-167~212). Shōzen's citation is verbatim.

62. See *Man'anpō,* chapter 15 (*KS,* pp. 460–463, XV-177-190).
63. See *Man'anpō,* chapter 15 (*KS,* p. 466, XV-202-203).
64. This is explicitly articulated by former emperor Hanazono when commenting on a passage from the *Zhongyang* 中庸 (Focusing the Familiar): 但君子素其位行，[不願乎其外]. 貧賤者素貧賤行、富貴者素富貴行. 是内径所謂先世之宿業、於外典之説謂命者也. "However, 'a true gentleman from the beginning (accordingly) conducts himself from this status. A poor and base person from the beginning conducts himself poorly and basely. A rich and noble person from the beginning conducts himself richly and nobly.' This is what the inner teachings [Buddhism] call the immutable karma from previous lives, and the outer teachings [Chinese writings] call destiny." *Hanazono tennō shinki,* Genkō 4 (1324).6.24.
65. In the *Ton'ishō,* following a section listing various symptoms and signs that would alert one as to whether an infant might die soon or would have a long or a short life, Shōzen drew a broader lesson about length of lifespan. He noted such examples as Confucius' talented disciple Yanhui, who, though brilliant, had died young, his promise unfulfilled, like a plum blossom scattered before the end of spring. Not dissimilarly, depending upon their inherent nature 性, some infants will have long lives and others will have short ones: *Ton'ishō,* chapter 35 (*KS,* p. 538, XVI-90-91).
66. *Man'anpō,* chapter 5 (*KS,* pp. 106–119, V-2-52); *Man'anpō,* index (*KS,* p. 5–6, M-20-22).
67. *Beiji qianjin yaofang,* chapter 23, pp. 427–428.
68. *Taiping shenghui fang,* chapters 24 and 25.
69. See *Shengji zonglu,* chapter 18 (pp. 439–472).
70. Compare *Shengji zonglu,* chapter 18 (p. 450), and *Man'anpō,* chapter 5 (*KS,* p. 111, V-19).
71. Compare *Shengji zonglu,* chapter 18 (pp. 455–456), and *Man'anpō,* chapter 5 (*KS,* p. 113, V-28).
72. Compare *Shengji zonglu,* chapter 18 (p. 467), and *Man'anpō,* chapter 5 (*KS,* p. 115, V-35).
73. Compare *Shengji zonglu,* chapter 18 (p. 460), and *Man'anpō,* chapter 5 (*KS,* p. 114, V-32).
74. *Hejiju fang,* chapter 1 (pp. 148–149, 150–151), *Man'anpō,* chapter 5 (*KS,* pp. 118–119, V-48-50).
75. *Man'anpō,* chapter 5 (*KS,* pp. 109–110, V-14-15; pp. 112–113, V-26-27; p. 113, V-30).
76. *Man'anpō,* chapter 5 (*KS,* p. 116, V-42). See also *Sanyin fang,* chapter 15 (p. 214).

Chapter 5 Warfare, Wound Medicine, and Song Medical Knowledge

1. For the political background, see Andrew Edmund Goble, *Kenmu: Go-Daigo's Revolution,* and Jeffrey P. Mass, "Of Hierarchy and Authority at the End of Kamakura." On the exigencies and rhythms of fourteenth-century warfare, see Thomas Conlan, *State of War: The Violent Order of Fourteenth-Century Japan.* For Hōjō deaths, see, for example, Helen Craig McCullough, trans., *The Taiheiki: A Chronicle of Medieval Japan,* pp. 266–272, 292–301, 310–311; and the Ōmi no kuni Banba shuku Rengeji kakō chō (*KI,* 42:32137), a register of the 430 Hōjō and their close supporters, aged between fourteen and sixty-four, who took their own lives en masse outside Kyoto on the seventh day of the fifth month of 1333.
2. The oldest extant version of this appears to be a sixteenth-century transcription of a copy made by three people in 1395 of an original compiled in 1356 or 1357. I wish to express my thanks to the late Mr. Sōda Hajime for his generosity in allowing me to photograph his personal copy of this in the spring of 1994. This, and the bulk of Mr. Sōda's collection focusing on the history of pharmacology in Japan, is now housed at the International Research Center for Japanese Studies in Kyoto. See Kokusai Nihon Bunka Kenkyū Sentā, 2001.
3. There is no further information on Norizane, although he may be an ancestor of the Tominokōji Michiyoshi (Tsūkei), whose connection with medical activity is noted for 1452: Shinmura Taku, *Nihon iryō shakaishi no kenkyū,* p. 116.
4. See Karl Friday, *Hired Swords: The Rise of Private Warrior Power in Early Japan.*
5. For a survey of pre-fourteenth-century warfare, see William Wayne Farris, *Heavenly Warriors: The Evolution of Japan's Military, 500–1300.*
6. See Karl Friday, "What a Difference a Bow Makes: The Rules of War in Early Medieval Japan."
7. See Jeffrey P. Mass, *Yoritomo and the Founding of the First Bakufu,* pp. 141 ff.
8. See Thomas Conlan, *In Little Need of Divine Intervention.*
9. On the multifaceted aspects of military force in the medieval period, see Conlan, *State of War,* and Karl F. Friday, *Samurai, Warfare and the State in Early Medieval Japan.* See also H. Paul Varley, *Warriors of Japan as Depicted in the War Tales,* for portrayals of warriors and fighting styles over time.
10. See *Taiheiki,* chapter 18 (vol. 2, pp. 244, 246). See also Varley, *Warriors of Japan as Depicted in the War Tales,* pp. 201–205.
11. See *Taiheiki,* chapter 26 (vol. 3, p. 14), noting that "over 500 troops" who had fallen into a freezing river were in pain for four to five days even after being given warm clothes, medicines, and having their wounds tended.

12. For example, see *Taiheiki,* chapter 17 (vol. 2, pp. 214–215, 236).
13. For the first reference to a spear, see Genkō 4 (1334).1.10 Soga Otsubōmaru (Takamitsu) dai Keitō Michitame teoi chūmon (*KI,* 42:32830; in *NBI-To,* 1:37 as Soga Otsubōmaru dai Shami Dōi kassen teoi chūmon). For examples of these other weapons, see *Taiheiki,* respectively chapters 8 (vol. 1, p. 263), chapter 7 (vol. 1, p. 221) and chapter 30 (vol. 3, p. 160), chapter 3 (vol. 1, p. 118), chapter 7 (vol. 1, p. 219), and chapter 7 (vol. 1, pp. 222–223).
14. This was first made explicit in a directive of Emperor Go-Daigo: see Genkō 3 (1333).4 Go-Daigo tennō rinji kotogaki an (*KI,* 41:32124). The policy outlasted Go-Daigo and his cause and became the standard of all military leaders thereafter.
15. On *gunchūjō,* see Urushibara Tōru, *Chūsei gunchūjō to sono sekai.* Neither registers of injuries nor battle service reports were new in the 1330s. *Azuma kagami,* Jōkyū 3 (1221).6.18 refers to records of people who received wounds or who were killed on specific days and in specific battles. Urushibara (p. 145, note 7) suggests that the first *gunchūjō* is the Kōan 5 (1282).2 Hishijima Tokinori gunchūjō (*KI,* 19:14538). However, the larger point is that these reports suddenly became ubiquitous in the 1330s.
16. In one document, a warrior notes that his loyal service in a recent battle consisted of having been shot high up on the right hip and being cut on the left forearm. See Rekiō 3 (1340).3.23 Okamoto Takahiro gunchūjō utsushi (*NBI-Ka,* 2:1101).
17. A report dated 1336.6.13 submitted by Kōno Michimori, for instance, details the casualties suffered by a contingent from Iyo Province in a week of fighting (1336.6.5, 6.6, and 6.11) around Mt. Hiei, outside the capital of Kyoto. Michimori records injuries to twenty-seven people: shot through from the left cheek to the right ear; pierced above the right nipple, breast, and left cheek, and shot in four other places; shot in the neck bone; shot through from beneath the right eye to below the ear; shot through the right arm; shot in the right shin; shot below the right armpit; shot through the top of the right foot; shot in the left armpit; shot through the right shin; pierced through the left shin; shot in the left shin; shot in the right arm; shot in the top of the right foot; shot through the left armpit; shot in the left thigh; shot in the right shoulder; shot in the right foot; shot in the right shoulder; shot in the right foot; shot in the right thigh; shot in the right thigh; shot in the right thigh; shot in the left knee; shot in the left thigh; shot in the left thigh; shot in the right shoulder; shot in the right shin; shot in the left shin. See Kenmu 3 (1336).6.13 Shami Zenkei (Kōno Michimori) teoi chūmon utsushi (*NBI-Ch,* 1:375).
18. For family injuries over time, see Kenmu 4 (1337).7 Soga Sadamitsu gunchūjō an (*NBI-To,* 1:332), noting eight people who had received arrow

wounds to right shoulder, left thigh, right neck bone, hips, below the right eye, right shoulder, below the left ear and to the sole of the right foot; and Kenmu 4 (1337).8.23 Soga Sadamitsu gunchūjō (*NBI-To,* 1:338), noting three people who had received a deep arrow wound to the right shoulder and arrow wounds to left thigh and left shoulder.

19. There are exceptions. *Taiheiki,* chapter 22 (vol. 2, p. 371), while not a battle report, notes a warrior who died three days after an arrowhead had lodged in the shoulder. Conlan, *State of War,* p. 26, notes an instance where one rescued warrior succumbed to seven sword and arrow wounds that evening and another instance where a warrior, wounded in the shoulder, lingered until he reached home a week later and then died. Parenthetically, while Conlan remarks that "many of the seriously wounded died shortly after battle because medical technology was primitive," and we must acknowledge that contemporary wound medicine had its limitations, the failure of wounded to survive might equally be attributed to the severity of the trauma.

20. For more detailed examination of weapons and injuries, see Anthropological Society of Japan, *Medieval Japanese Skeletons from the Burial Site at Zaimokuza, Kamakura City;* Myra Shackley, "Arms and the Men: 14th Century Japanese Swordsmanship Illustrated by Skeletons from Zaimokuza"; Anthony Karasulas, "Zaimokuza Reconsidered: The Forensic Evidence, and Classical Japanese Swordsmanship." Shackley and Karasulas reach different conclusions on the type of weapons used to inflict injuries and on the social and military status of the combatants involved. Thomas Conlan, *State of War,* pp. 43–69; Thomas Conlan, "Nambokuchō ki kassen no ichi kōsatsu: Sen shishō kara mita tokushitsu," p. 431, table 5; Shakadō Mitsuhiro, "Nanbokuchō ki kassen ni okeru senjō." Conlan and Shakadō use different criteria for classifying head and torso injuries, and they interpret differently such things as the effectiveness of weapons, fatality rates, and reasons for the relative scarcity of upper body wounds compared to wounds to the extremities.

21. We have references to, for instance, thirteen wounds in one battle; five wounds (forehead, left arm, right eyebrow, right hip, right thigh); a person cut and shot in eleven places, another in five places; cut and shot in seven places, wounded in three places (stomach, chest, right knee); and two people each wounded twice (right thigh and right armpit, head and right shoulder). See Rekiō 3 (1340).3 Takuma Munetada gunchūjō (*NBI-Ky,* 2:1497); Kōei 2 (1343).8 Kikkawa Tsuneaki gunchūjō (*NBI-Ch,* 2:1289); Kan'ō 2 (1351).8 Nejime Kiyonari gunchūjō (*NBI-Ky,* 3:3174); Bunwa 3 (1354).3. Takebe [Nejime] Kiyonari, Kiyoari gunchūjō utsushi (*NBI-Ky,* 3:3669).

22. In one case a warrior reports being shot three times in little over a year: in the left knee, the middle finger of the left hand, and the right anklebone. See Kōei 3 (1344).2 Beppu Michizane gunchūjō utsushi (*NBI-Ka,* 2:1480).

23. In the report cited in the preceding note, the writer notes that an arrowhead remained lodged in his right anklebone and that he was near death several times but remained in camp directing his forces. It seems that the wound was not permanently disabling, since some seventeen years later we find the shōgun thanking him for his battle efforts. Enbun 5 (1360), intercalary 4.9 Ashikaga Yoshiakira mikan mikyōsho (*Shinpen Saitama kenshi shiryōhen* 5 *chūsei* 1, doc. 433, p. 310).
24. For example, in one battle in 1338, out of 254 combatants in one contingent, 6 were wounded by arrows and 14 were killed. See Kenmu 5 (1338).3 Matsura tō tōshi kassen kōmyō utsushi (*NBI-Ky,* 1:1161).
25. Concerns about the accuracy of figures in sources have been expressed for some time. See Sir George Sansom, *A History of Japan to 1334,* inter alia; Sansom, *A History of Japan, 1334–1615,* pp. 119–124. More recently, see Farris, *Heavenly Warriors,* pp. 97–98, 269–273, 291–292, 300–302, 316–319, 324–327, 333–334; and Conlan, *In Little Need of Divine Intervention,* pp. 261–264.
26. See respectively, *Kasuga gongen genkie* (1982), p. 13; *Zenkunen kassen ekotoba,* pp. 38–39; *Heiji monogatari emaki,* p. 90; *Zenkunen kassen ekotoba,* p. 37; *Kasuga gongen genkie* (1963), pp. 44–45, 84; *Gosannen kassen ekotoba,* p. 50.
27. *Mutsu waki* speaks of troops suffering 13 dead and 158 wounded and their commander providing care for them, but it provides no further details: See H. C. McCullough (tr.), "A Tale of Mutsu," pp. 196–197. The *Hōgen monogatari* speaks of someone trying unsuccessfully to treat an arrow wound to the neck by applying moxibustion to the mouth of the wound: See William Wilson (tr.), *Hōgen Monogatari: Tale of the Disorder in Hōgen,* pp. 46–47. In another case, moxibustion was used to revive a warrior who had nearly drowned: *Azuma kagami,* Jōkyū 3 (1221).6.14 (see also William McCullough, "The *Azuma Kagami* Account of the Shōkyū War," p. 127).
28. See respectively *Gosannen kassen ekotoba,* p. 19; *Gosannen kassen ekotoba,* p. 20; *Ashibiki emaki,* black and white plate 13.
29. *Azuma kagami* records that in order to execute a person, Shibuya Takashige had to hold his sword in only one hand, since he had been wounded in the arm about twelve days earlier: See *Azuma kagami,* Juei 3/Genryaku 1(1184).2.2; also Minoru Shinoda, *The Founding of the Kamakura Shogunate, 1180–1185,* p. 248. *Taiheiki* chapter 17 (vol. 2, p. 221) provides the example of Takeda Gorō, who, because cuts to his fingers had made it impossible for him to hold a sword, strapped a wooden sword to his right chest and went into battle.
30. The *Taiheiki,* chapter 16 (vol. 2, p. 146) notes that one Wada Takanori was unable to see properly as a result of the combined effect of wounds from a previous battle that had not healed and the movement of his horse.

31. *Azuma kagami* and *Hōgen monogatari* state that Ōba Kageyoshi, whose knee was pierced by an arrow in the Hōgen Incident of 1156, was rendered virtually incapable of walking for the rest of his life. William Wilson (tr.), *Hōgen Monogatari: Tale of the Disorder in Hōgen,* pp. 42–43; and *Azuma kagami,* Bunji 5 (1189).6.30. The *Hōgen monogatari* entry notes that Kageyoshi was shot while having paused, and that had he not been physically carried off the battlefield by his brother, he would certainly have had his head taken by the enemy. Later in life, Kageyoshi remembered that knowledge of opponents' archery techniques had enabled him to maneuver so that he was shot in the knee rather than in the body. See *Azuma kagami,* Kenkyū 2 (1191).8.1; cited also in Friday, *Samurai, Warfare and the State in Early Medieval Japan,* p. 109. My thanks to Professor Motoki Yasuo of Kyoto University for bringing this example to my attention.
32. *Shasekishū,* 2.4 (pp. 96–98; Robert Morrell, *Sand and Pebbles,* pp. 106–108).
33. *Azuma kagami,* Kenchō 6 (1254).5.5.
34. Kenji 1 (1275).10.28 Kii no kuni Ategawa no shō Kamimura hyakushō ra gonjōjō (*KI,* 16:12076). See also Nakamura Ken, "Jitō hihō to katakana gonjōjō."
35. Shōka 3 (1259).1 Futadokoro jingū tsukai ra mōshijō (*KI,* 11:8341).
36. *Shasekishū,* 2.4 (pp. 96–98; Morrell, *Sand and Pebbles,* pp. 106–108). Morrell translates *fukuchū,* within the abdomen, as "lungs," which would seem to make sense for an injury to the windpipe.
37. For the story, see *Konjaku monogatari,* 29:25 (*Nihon koten bungaku zensho,* vol. 4, p. 403, n. 16; *NKBT,* vol. 5, p. 179, n. 6). For a discussion of Dried Infant, see Andrew Edmund Goble, "War and Injury: The Emergence of Wound Medicine in Medieval Japan," pp. 321–324.
38. Shinmura Taku, *Nihon iryō shakaishi no kenkyū,* p. 109, citing Kenkyū 9 (1198).5 Kasuga kannushi Nakatomi Sukeaki ge (*KI,* 2:982).
39. For the tooth puller, see *Shasekishū,* 8.23 (pp. 361–362; Morrell, *Sand and Pebbles,* pp. 229–230). For the eye specialist, see *Yamai no sōshi,* pp. 89–91. The text for the scene notes,

    > Recently a man in Yamato Province was lamenting the slight loss of vision in his eye. Just then someone appeared at the gate, and when asked who he was said that "I am a doctor who treats ailments of the eye." The master of the house invited him in, thinking that this must be help from the gods and Buddhas. The man raised the eye-[lid], had a look, and noting that it would be best to treat it with a needle, applied the needle. He then left, saying that it will be better soon. After that it became increasingly difficult to see, and in the end he lost the sight in one eye.

For further exploration of this scroll and the *Scroll of Gross Afflictions,* see Andrew Edmund Goble, "Images of Illness: Interpreting the Medieval *Scrolls of Afflictions.*"

40. For useful surveys of court physicians and the organization of medical services, see Shinmura, *Kodai iryō kanjinsei no kenkyū;* Yamada Shigemasa, *Ten'i no rekishi.*
41. For a brief look at the court physicians and their descendents recruited by the Kamakura *bakufu,* see Higuchi Seitarō, "*Azumi kagami* o chūshin toshite mita Kamakura no ishi."
42. See Hattori Toshirō, *Nara jidai igakushi no kenkyū,* pp. 100–102, 193, 196; and *Heian jidai igakushi no kenkyū,* pp. 228–229. For comment on volume 18 of the *Ishinpō,* see Shinmura Taku, *Nihon iryō shakaishi no kenkyū,* p. 111; Nagai Chū, "*Ishinpō* o chūshin to seru Nihon kodai no gunjin geka."
43. *Ton'ishō,* chapter 24 (*KS,* p. 408, XII-62). The formula is taken from the *Hejiju fang* (see *Kankoku zōkō Taiping Hejiju fang,* vol. 2, p. 555), but the reference to re-growing flesh in the case of a wound is not found in that text.
44. *Ton'ishō,* chapter 40 (*KS,* p. 605, XIX-41-42).
45. See *Hejiju fang,* chapter 8, pp. 532–564; *Puji benshi fang,* chapter 6, pp. 239–241; *Shizhai baiyi xuanfang,* chapter 12, pp. 383–387.
46. *Man'anpō,* chapter 24 (*KS,* p. 689, XXIV-89).
47. *Man'anpō,* chapter 62 (*KS,* p. 1704, LXII-30).
48. *Man'anpō,* chapter 24 (*KS,* p. 676, XXIV-37). Parenthetically, *Azuma kagami,* Shōka 2 (1258).16, 17, 18 notes a case where the tip of an arrow that had been used to shoot a person to death had been daubed with poison.
49. See *Yuyaoyuan fang,* vol. 8 (vol. 2, p. 499–503). The five formulas for treating unbearable pain, treating internal bleeding after a fall from a high place, unbearable pain from cuts and breaks, pain, and constipation and lack of urination, have been taken en bloc from the work.
50. *Gogumaiki,* Meitoku 3 (1392).2.1, 2.3, 2.4 (3.110, 111), noting that the famous wound physician Rakuami, a house vassal of the warrior Uramatsu Sukeyasu 裏松資康, had been called to treat a lady of the imperial household who had been slashed with a sword by the emperor.
51. *Kinsō ryōjishō,* postscript, preface.
52. *Kihō,* section 19 (p. 275).
53. *Ton'ishō,* chapter 45 (*KS,* p. 678, XXII-41-42). My initial reference, and the identification of the Kawatsu Lay Priest as Itō Sukechika, is from Ishihara Akira, "Kajiwara Shōzen no shōgai to sono chosho," p. 1742.
54. See Shibata, *Hōryūji shozō Iyaku chōzai koshō,* item 34, pp. 31, 48.
55. *Kihō,* sections 2 (p. 259), 4 (p. 267), 5 (p. 263), 9 (pp. 266, 267), 17 (p. 274), 19 (p. 277), 24 (p. 279), and 28 (p. 281).

56. *Kihō,* section 35 (p. 286). *Kihō* provides recipes for this life-preserving medicine: *kuroyaki,* also known as *fushi no kusuri* in two other sections, *Kihō* section 38 (p. 288) and *Kihō* section 4 (p. 262). In the latter case, the author notes that if it is vomited up, the person will die, but if not, the person will live.
57. For "*my oral transmissions,*" see *Kihō* section 10 (p. 270). For unspecified oral transmissions, see *Kihō* sections 1 (pp. 256, 257) and 4 (p. 261).
58. *Kihō,* section 10 (p. 268). See also "*Kihō* states," section 35 (p. 286).
59. *Kihō,* section 39 (p. 289).
60. *Kinsō ryōjishō,* section 55.
61. *Kinsō ryōjishō,* sections 11, 12, 15, 20, 21, 44 (twice). Section 11 refers to a Nanbu (fu) Lay Priest 南部入道, who may be the same Nanfu Lay Priest of sections 21 and 44.
62. *Kinsō ryōjishō,* sections 15, 16, 44, 55.
63. See chapter 3 in the present volume; and, for example, *Ton'ishō* chapter 12 (*KS,* p. 223, VII-9).
64. *Yeshi luyan fang,* pp. 355–356.
65. Karl Friday, *Samurai, Warfare, and the State in Early Medieval Japan,* pp. 71–72.
66. *Ton'ishō,* chapter 21 (*KS,* pp. 370–71, X-159~160); Ibid. (X-160~161).
67. *Ton'ishō,* chapter 29 (*KS,* p. 455, XIII-141~142); Ibid. (XIII-142).
68. *Ton'ishō,* chapter 29 (*KS,* p. 458, XIII-153~155). The reference to "having been opened by a man" could be taken as applying to injuries caused by having intercourse for the first time or from undergoing forcible intercourse. However, given that the term "opened" or "to open" seems to have been a colloquial medieval term for sexual intercourse in general, I have interpreted the comment in this broader sense. For an example of the use of "opened," in this case a derogatory and accusatory reference to "mother opening" 母開, see Kenchō 1 (1249).7.23 Kantō gechijō (*KI,* 10:7093).
69. *Ton'ishō,* chapter 33 (*KS,* p. 512, XV-95); Ibid. (XV-95~96); Ibid. (XV-96).
70. *Ton'ishō,* chapter 24 (*KS,* p. 397, XII-17~20). As noted in chapter 4 of this volume, one of the injunctions in *Ton'ishō* for *rai* patients undergoing one specific treatment is that they are to avoid certain types of foods, not lock eyes with someone suffering the same affliction, and not share lodging with a woman who is experiencing menstruation: See *Ton'ishō,* chapter 34 (*KS,* pp. 526–527, XVI-42~45) for foods; Ibid. (XVI-42) on human contact.
71. *Ton'ishō,* chapter 24 (*KS,* p. 400, XII-31~33).
72. *Ton'ishō,* chapter 24 (*KS,* pp. 403–405, XII-44~52). Cloud Mother Ointment became one of the most touted medicines of the medieval era. For mention of it as one of two noted ointments, see *Sekiso ōrai,* p. 609.

73. See the quite short *Ton'ishō,* chapter 23 (*KS*, pp. 385–392, XI-50~78).
74. *Ton'ishō,* chapter 27 (*KS,* pp. 425–426, XIII-24~25).
75. *Ton'ishō,* chapter 29 (*KS,* p. 452, XIII-131~132).
76. *Ton'ishō,* chapter 31 (*KS,* p. 475, XIV-61~62); Ibid. (*KS,* p. 483, XIV-96).
77. *Ton'ishō,* chapter 32 (*KS,* pp. 496–497, XV-29~30, 32~33).
78. *Ton'ishō,* chapter 29 (*KS,* p. 457, XIII-149~150).
79. *Ton'ishō,* chapter 33 (*KS,* pp. 512–513, XV-95~96, 98).
80. *Ton'ishō,* chapter 36 (*KS,* pp. 555–556, XVII-36~37); Ibid. (*KS,* pp. 560–561, XVII-53~57).
81. *Ton'ishō,* chapter 21 (*KS,* p. 364, X-135); Ibid. (*KS,* p. 365, X-137~138); Ibid. (*KS,* p. 364, X-135~136); Ibid. (*KS,* p. 368, X-151).
82. *Ton'ishō,* chapter 27 (*KS,* p. 426, XIII-25).
83. *Ton'ishō,* chapter 29 (*KS,* p. 455, XIII-142~143).
84. *Ton'ishō,* 32 (*KS,* p. 500, XV-46); Ibid. (*KS,* pp. 496–497, XV-32~33).
85. *Kihō,* section 41 (pp. 291–292).
86. For these latter, see *Kihō,* sections 1 (p. 257), 9 (p. 266), 10 (p. 267), 10 (p. 268), and *Kinsō ryōjishō,* section 3.
87. *Kihō,* section 30 (p. 284).
88. *Kinsō ryōjishō,* section 12.
89. *Kihō,* section 41 (pp. 291–292). The items are musk, aloes, cassia, Chinese licorice, turmeric, ginseng, cardamom, fossil bones, snake bones, white sandalwood, cloves, Burmese rosewood, *kutsuriki,* Borneo camphor tree, Chinese costus, white atractylodes (百朮), white atractylodes (オケラ), fennel, ash from the skull of a white dog, powder of the skull of a chestnut-colored horse, pine resin, oil, boar oil, ash of clam, Rehmannia root, mulberry seed, *sokuzu,* gall of mountain hawk-eagle, oil of bear, bark of mountain apricot, and three unidentified items: Western Sea Branch 西海枝, Tiger Vermilion Fragrance 虎丹香, and Ear Not Think 耳不思 (if there had been some jumbling and transcription errors, then one of the latter might be 虎耳草 Saxifrage).

Epilogue: Engaging Song Medical Knowledge

1. See Kenneth G. Zysk, *Asceticism and Healing in Ancient India: Medicine in the Buddhist Monastery.*

GLOSSARY

Avatamsaka Sutra 華厳経
Beiji jiu fang 備急灸方
Beiji qianjin yaofang 備急千金要方
Bencaojing 本草経
Bian Que 扁鵲
Chanbao fang 産宝方
Changxin 常心
Chao Yuanfang 巣元方
Chen Shiwen 陳師文
Chen Yan 陳言
Chen Ziming 陳自明
chigo hoshi 児干
Chōboji 長母寺
Chongguang buzhu Huangdi neijing suwen 重広補注黄帝内経素問
Chōsei ryōyōhō 長生療養方
Chu Yushi 初虞世
Cihong 慈洪
Daguan bencao 大観本草
Daidō ruijūhō 大同類聚方
Daihatsu nehan gyō 大般涅槃経
Daishi *seng* 大食僧
Daoguang 道廣
Daomiao 道妙
Dayiju fang 大医局方

Dazaifu 大宰府
denshibyō 伝屍病
Denshibyō nijūgo hō 伝屍病二十五方
Dōshō 道生
Eisei hiyōshō 衛生秘要抄
Eison 叡尊
Enni Ben'en 円爾弁円
Ennin 円仁
Fengke jiyan mingfang 風科集験名方
Fukane Sukebito 深根輔仁
Fukudenpō 福田方
funaigai in 不内外因
Furen daquan liangfang 婦人大全良方
Gahō 我宝
Give-Five General 与五将軍
gōbyō 業病
Go-Daigo 後醍醐
Gokurakuji 極楽寺
Gokurakuji letter 極楽寺殿御消息
Go-Shirakawa 後白河
Gotai miwakeshū 五体身分集
Great Teacher of Mt. Kōya 高野大師
gunchūjō 軍忠状
Guo Tan 郭坦
Hakata 博多
Hakozaki Shrine 箱崎神社
Hanazono花園
Hangzhou 杭州
Hanzhang 漢章
Hejiju fang 和剤局方
hinin 非人
Hōjō Naritoki 北条業時
Hōjō Sadatoki 北条貞時

Hōjō Shigetoki 北条重時
Hōjō Takatoki 北条高時
Hōjō Tokimune 北条時宗
Hōjō Tokiyori 北条時頼
Hokiron 補気論
Hokkekyō, Myōhō renge kyō 法華経 , 妙法蓮華経
Honzō iroha shō 本草色葉鈔
Honzō wamyō 本草和名
Hōryūji 法隆寺
Huangdi 黄帝
Huangdi neijing suwen 黄帝内経素問
Huiqing 恵清
Huoren shizheng fang houji 活人事証方後集
Idanshō 医談抄
Ikkyū 一休
Ippen 一遍
Ippen shōnin eden 一遍上人絵伝
Iryakushō 医略抄
Ishinpō 医心方
Issaikyō 一切経
Itō Sukechika 伊藤祐親
Iyaku chōzai koshō 医薬調剤古抄
Jianyi fanglun 簡易方論
Jiayou buzhu bencao 嘉祐補注本草
Jingui yaolüe fanglun 金匱要略方論
Jingxiao chanbao 経効産宝
Jingyi fang 精義方
Jingzhilu 敬止録
Jisshō 實照
Jisshō-in 實相院
Jivaka 耆婆
Jōjin 成尋
Jōshun 定舜

Jōtenji 承天寺
Kaibao xinxiang ding bencao 開宝新詳定本草
Kajiwara Shōzen 梶原性全
Kakujō 覚浮
Kamakura 鎌倉
Kanazawa Bunko 金沢文庫
Kanezawa Sadaaki 金沢貞顕
Kanezawa Sanetoki 金沢実時
karabune 唐舟
karamono 唐物
kawaramono 河原者
Kawatsu Lay Priest 河津入道
Kazō hihō/Jiacang mifang 家蔵秘方
Kegon kyō 華厳経
Kenchōji 建長寺
Ken'i 兼意
Kenninji 建仁寺
Keyong fang 可用方
Kihō 鬼法
Kinsō ryōjishō 金瘡療治抄
Kissa yōjōki 喫茶養生記
Kōjishō 香字抄
Koremune Tomotoshi 惟宗具俊
Kōshū 光宗
Kōyakushō 香薬抄
Kōyōshō 香要抄
Kujō Michiie 九条道家
Langyuan *fang* 朗元房
Lanxi Daolong 蘭渓道隆
Li Minshou 黎民壽
Liu Xinfu 劉信甫
Maka shikan (Ch. *Mohe ziguan*) 摩訶止観
Man'anpō 万安方

Minamoto Sanetomo 源実朝
Mingji Chujun 明極楚俊
Mingtangtu 明堂図
Mingtangtu jing 明堂図経
Mingzhou 明州
Mujū Ichien 無住 一円
Munakata Shrine 宗像神社
Myōan Eisai 明庵栄西
Myōnin 明忍
Nagai Munehide 長井宗秀
Nagai Sadahide 長井貞秀
Nanfu Lay Priest 南浮入道
Nichiren 日蓮
Nikaidō 二階堂
Nikaidō Yukifuji 二階堂行藤
Ningbo 寧波
Ninshō 忍性
Puji benshi fang 普済本事方
qi 気
Qianjin fang 千金方
Qingzhuo ōshō 清拙和尚
Rai 癩
Rakuami 楽阿弥
Rencun Sunshi zhibing huofa mifang 仁存孫氏治病活法秘方
Renki 蓮基
Rennyo 連如
Ritsu 律
Saidaiji 西大寺
Sanyin fang 三因方
Shanghan huorenshu 傷寒活人書
Shanghan lun 傷寒論
Shasekishū 沙石集
Shennong 神農

Shenghui fang 聖恵方
Shengji fang 聖済方
Shengji zonglu 聖済総録
Shibian liangfang 十便良方
Shichirō "Boat-Captain" Funagashira 七郎船頭
Shingon 眞言
Shinsarugaku ki 新猿楽記
Shizhai baiyi xuanfang 是斎百一選方
Shōchū hō 掌中方
Shōfukuji 聖福寺
Shōmi kagami 賞味鏡
Shōmyōji 称名寺
Shōni Sukeyoshi 少弐資能
Storax Pill 蘇合香
Su 蘇
Sun Rencun 孫仁存
Sun Simiao 孫思邈
Sun Yunxian 孫允賢
Suwen jing 素問経
Taiping huimin Hejiju fang 太平恵民和剤局方
Taiping Shenghui fang 太平聖恵方
Taiping yulan 太平御覧
Taira Kiyomori 平清盛
Tanba Masatada 丹波雅忠
Tanba Yasuyori 丹波康頼
Tanba Yukinaga 丹波行長
Tendai 天台
Tōdaiji 東大寺
Tōfukuji 東福寺
Tominokōji Norizane 富小路範實
Tong Zhenzi 通眞子
Tong Zhenzi maijue 通眞子脉訣
Ton'ishō 頓医抄

Tōtōmi Lay Priest 遠江入道
Tripitika 大蔵経
Tsūken nyūdō zōsho mokuroku 通憲入道蔵書目録
Uritsu no kan 宇律官
Waike jingyao 外科精要
Waitai miyao fang 外台秘要方
Wake 和気
Wake Tadakage 和気忠景
Wang, Ms. 王氏
Wang Huaiyin 王懐隠
Wang Qiu 王璆
Wang Shuhe 王叔和
Wang Shuhe maijue 王叔和脉訣
Wang Shuo 王碩
Wanshou Chansi 万壽禅寺
Wei Xian 魏峴
Weishi jiacang fang 魏氏家蔵方
Xie Guoming 謝国明
Xu Guozhen 許国禎
Xu Shuwei 許叔微
Xu yijian fang 続易簡方
Yakumei ruijū 薬名類聚
Yakushō 薬抄
Yakushushō 薬種抄
Yamai no sōshi 病の草紙
Yan Yonghe 厳用和
Yang Rong 楊榮
Yang Tan 楊倓
Yangsheng biyong fang 養生必用方
Yangshi jiacang fang 楊氏家蔵方
Yanshi jisheng fang 厳氏済生方
Ye Dalian 葉大廉
Yeshi luyan fang 葉氏録験方

Yi, Presider 義首座
Yifang jicheng 医方集成
Yijian fang 易簡方
Yishuo 医説
Yōketsushō 要穴抄
Youyou xinshu 幼幼新書
Yu Fu 俞跗
Yueguang 楽廣
Yuyaoyuan fang 御薬院方
Zan Yin 昝殷
Zatsuzatsu hō/Zaza fang 雑々方
Zhang, Ms. 張氏
Zhang Guang'an 張光安
Zhang Zhongjing 張仲景
Zhenzhong fang 枕中方
Zhiguang 智光
Zhiyi 智顗
Zhu Gong 朱肱
Zhubing yuanhou zonglun 諸病源候總論

BIBLIOGRAPHY

Note: Unless otherwise specified, the place of publication for Chinese titles is Beijing and for Japanese titles is Tokyo.

Primary Sources

Ashibiki emaki 足引絵巻. In *Kassen emaki* 合戦絵巻. Ed. Miya Tsugio 宮次男. Kadokawa Shoten 角川書店, 1977.

Azuma kagami 吾妻鏡. In *KT,* vols. 32–33.

Beiji qianjin yaofang 備急千金要方. By Sun Simiao 孫思邈. Renmin Weisheng Chubanshe 人民衛生出版社, 1982.

Bingashū 岷峨集. By Sesson Yūbai 雪村友梅. In *Gozan bungaku zenshū* 五山文学全集, vol. 1: 519–566. Ed. Uemura Kankō 上村観光. Kyoto 京都: Shibunkaku Shuppan 思文閣出版, 1973 reprint.

Chōsei ryōyōhō 長生療養方. By Renki 蓮基. In *ZGR,* vol. 30.2: 143–174.

Chūsei hōsei shiryō shū (*CHSS*) 中世法制史料集, vol. 1. Ed. Ikeuchi Yoshisuke 池内義資 and Satō Shin'ichi 佐藤進一. Iwanami Shoten 岩波書店, 1955.

Daidō ruijūhō 大同類聚方. By Izumo no Hirosada 出雲広貞 and Abe no Manao 阿倍真直. In Maki Sachiko 槙佐知子 *Zen'yaku seikai Daidō ruijūhō* 全訳精解大同類聚方. Shinsensha 新泉社, 1992.

Denshibyō nijūgo hō 伝死病二十五方. By Gahō 我宝. In *ZGR,* vol. 31.1: 264–275.

Eisei hiyōshō 衛生秘要抄. By Tanba Yukinaga 丹波行長. In *ZGR,* vol. 31.1: 205–218.

Fukudenpō 福田方. By Yūrin 有林. Kagaku Shoin 科学書院, 1987.

Fukutomi zōshi 福富草紙. In *Nihon emaki taisei* 日本絵巻大成, vol. 25. Ed. Komatsu Shigemi 小松茂美. Chūō Kōron Sha 中央公論社, 1979. Tr. in Virginia Skord, *Tales of Tears and Laughter.* Honolulu: University of Hawai'i Press, 1991.

Fumon'in Kyō Ron Shō So Goroku Jusho ra mokuroku 普門院経論章疎語録儒書等目録. In Shiraishi Kogetsu 白石虎月. Ed. *Tōfukuji shi* 東福寺誌: 381–395. Kyoto 京都: Shibunkaku Shuppan 思文閣主出版, 1979.

Furen daquan liangfang 婦人大全良方. By Chen Ziming 陳自明. In vol. 3-1 of *Wakoku Kanseki isho shūsei* 和刻漢籍医書集成. Ed. Kosoto Hiroshi 小曽戸洋. Entapuraizu エンタプライズ, 1989.

Genkō shakusho 元亨釋書. By Kokan Shiren 虎関師錬. In *KT,* vol. 31.

Gogumaiki 後愚昧記. By Sanjō Kintada 三条公忠. 4 vols. In *Dai Nihon kokiroku* 大日本古記録. Iwanami Shoten 岩波書店, 1980–1992.

Gokurakuji dono onshōsoku 極楽寺殿御消息. By Hōjō Shigetoki 北条重時. In *Chūsei seiji shakai shisō, jō* 中世政治社会思想上: 322–346. Ed. Ishii Susumu 石井進 et al. Iwanami Shoten 岩波書店, 1972. Translated in Carl Steenstrup, *Hōjō Shigetoki,* qv: 162–198.

Gokuraku Ritsuji shi 極楽律寺史. Vol. 1 *Chūsei kinsei hen* 中世近世編, vol. 2 *Chōkoku kōgei sekizō kenzōbutsu hen* 彫刻工芸石造建造物編. Ed. Ryōjusen Kan'ō'in Gokuraku Ritsuji 霊鷲山感応院極楽律寺編. Kamakura 鎌倉, 2003.

Gosannen kassen ekotoba 後三年合戦絵詞. *Nihon emaki taisei* 日本絵巻大成, vol. 15. Ed. Komatsu Shigemi 小松茂美. Chūō Kōron Sha 中央公論社, 1977.

Gotai miwakeshū 五体身分集. By Shōsai 生西. Microfilm hard copy of manuscript held in the library of Keiō Gijuku University 慶應義塾大学所蔵.

Gunsho ruijū (GR) 新校群書類従. Ed. Hanawa Hokinoichi 塙保己一. 24 vols. Naigai Shoseki Kabushiki Kaisha 内外書籍株式会社, 1931–1937.

Gyokuyō 玉葉. By Kujō Kanezane 九条兼実. 3 vols. Ed. Kokusho Sōsho Kankōkai 国書叢書刊行会. Meicho Kankōkai 名著刊行会, 1993.

Hanazono tennō shinki 花園天皇宸記. By Hanazono Tennō 花園天皇. 3 vols. In *Shiryō sanshū* 史料纂集, vols. 62, 66, 80. Zoku Gunsho Ruijū Kanseikai 続群書類従完成会, 1982–1986.

Heiji monogatari emaki 平治物語絵巻. In *Zoku Nihon emaki taisei* 続日本絵巻大成, vol. 17. Ed. Komatsu Shigemi 小松茂美. Chūō Kōron Sha 中央公論社, 1983.

Hejiju fang 和剤局方. See *Taiping huimin Hejiju fang.*

Hōgen monogatari 保元物語. Ed. Nagazumi Yasuaki 永積安明 and Shimada Isao 島田勇雄. In *NKBT,* vol. 31. Translated in William Wilson, *Hōgen*

Monogatari: Tale of the Disorder in Hōgen. Tokyo: Voyager's Press (for Monumenta Nipponica), 1966.

Honchō shojaku mokuroku 本朝書籍目録. In *GR,* vol. 21: 521–538.

Honzō iroha shō 本草色葉鈔. By Koremune Tomotoshi 惟宗具俊. Naikaku Bunko 内閣文庫, 1968.

Honzō wamyō 本草和名. By Fukane Sukebito 深根輔仁. In *ZGR,* vol. 30.2: 371–434.

Huoren shizheng fang houji 活人事証方後集. By Liu Xinfu 劉信甫. Taipei 台北: Xinwenfeng Chuban Gongsi 新文豊出版公司, 1987.

Idanshō 医談抄. By Koremune Tomotoshi 惟宗具俊. In *Idanshō* 医談抄 (*Denjō bungaku shiryō shūsei* 伝承文学資料集成 22). Ed. Minobe Shigekatsu 美濃部重克. Miyai Shoten 三弥井書店, 2006.

Ippen shōnin eden 一遍上人絵伝. In *Nihon no emaki* 日本の絵巻, vol. 20. Ed. Komatsu Shigemi 小松茂実. Chūō Kōronsha 中央公論社, 1988.

Ishinpō 医心方. By Tanba Yasuyori 丹波康頼. *Ishinpō: Nihon igaku sōsho katsujibon* 医心方日本医学叢書活字本. Osaka 大阪: Oriento Shuppansha オリエント出版社, 1991. See also Maki Sachiko 槇佐知子, *Zen'yaku seikai Ishinpō* 全訳精解医心方, Chikuma Shobō 筑摩書房, 1993–. Partial translations: 1/ Emil Hsia, Ilza Veith, Robert Geertsma, trans., *The Essentials of Medicine in Ancient China and Japan: Yasuyori Tanba's Ishinpō;* Leiden: Brill, 1986. 2/ Howard Levy and Ishihara Akira, trans., *The Tao of Sex: An Annotated Translation of the Twenty-Eighth Section of the Essence of Medical Prescriptions (Ishinpō*). Yokohama: Shibundō, 1968.

Iyaku chōzai koshō 医薬調剤古抄. In *Hōryūji shozō Iyaku chōzai koshō* 法隆寺所蔵医薬調剤古抄. Ed. Shibata Shōji 柴田承二. Hirokawa Shoten 廣川書店, 1997.

Jōrakuki 常楽記. In *GR,* vol. 22: 485–512.

Kamakura ibun komonjo hen (KI) 鎌倉遺文古文書編. Edited and compiled by Takeuchi Rizō 竹内理三. 42 volumes; plus 4 additional volumes and 5 index volumes. Tōkyōdō Shuppan 東京堂出版, 1971–1997.

Kamakura ibun munengō monjo mokuroku 鎌倉遺文無年号文書目録. Ed. Seno Seiichirō 瀬野精一郎. Tōkyōdō Shuppan 東京堂出版, 1993.

Kamakura shishi shiryō hen 2, 鎌倉市史史料編 *2.* Ed. Kamakura Shishi Hensan Iinkai 鎌倉市史編纂委員会. Yoshikawa Kōbunkan 吉川弘文館, 1956.

Kasuga gongen genkie (1963) 春日権現験記絵. In *Nihon emakimono zenshū* 日本絵巻物全集, vol. 15. Ed. Noma Seiroku 野間清六. Kadokawa Shoten 角川書店, 1963.

Kasuga gongen genkie (1982), *jō* 春日権現験記絵, 上. In *Zoku Nihon emaki taisei* 続日本絵巻大成, vol. 14. Ed. Komatsu Shigemi 小松茂美. Chūō Kōron Sha 中央公論社, 1982.

Keiran shūyōshū 渓嵐拾葉集. By Kōshū 光宗. *T.* 76, no. 2410.

Kihō 鬼法. By Tominokōji Norizane 富小路範實. In *Nihon eisei bunko* 日本衛生文庫, vol. 3. Ed. Miyake Hiizu 三宅秀 and Ōsawa Kenji 大澤謙二. Kyōiku Shinchō Kenkyūkai 教育新潮研究会, 1918. Repr. Nihon Tosho Sentā 日本図書センター, 1979.

Kinsō ryōjishō 金瘡療治. Anonymous manuscript (orig. compiled in fourteenth century), held in the Sōda Collection. See *Sōda bunko mokuroku shoseki hen* 宗田文庫目録書籍篇. Ed. Kokusai Nihon Bunka Kenkyū Sentā Sōda Bunko Mokuroku Henshū Iinkai 国際日本文化研究センター 宗田文庫目録編集委員会. Kyoto 京都: Kokusai Nihon Bunka Kenkyū Sentā 国際日本文化研究センター, 2001.

Kissa yōjōki 喫茶養生記. By Myōan Eisai 明庵栄西. In Furuta Shōkin 古田紹欽. *Eisai Kissa yōjō ki* 栄西喫茶養生記. Kōdansha 講談社, 2000.

Kōan yonnen ikoku onkitō ki 弘安四年異国御祈祷記. In *ZGR,* vol. 26.1: 176–186.

Kōjishō 香字抄. By Ken'i 兼意. In 1/ *Jūyō bunkazai* Kōjishō *(eiin bon)* 重要文化財 香字抄 (影印本). Ed. Koizumi Enjun 古泉圓順, Ōsaka 大阪: Takeda Kagaku Shinkō Zaidan 武田科学振興財団, 2007. 2/ *ZGR,* vol. 30.2: 467–540.

Kokon chomonjū 古今著聞集. By Tachibana Narisue 橘成季. 1/ Ed. Nagazumi Yasuaki 永積安明 and Shimada Isao 島田勇雄. In *NKBT,* vol. 84. 2/ In *KT,* vol. 19.

Kokushi taikei (KT) 新訂増補国史大系. Revised and enlarged edition. Ed. Kuroita Katsumi 黒板勝美. 60 vols. Yoshikawa Kōbunkan 吉川弘文館, 1964–67.

Konjaku monogatari 今昔物語. Ed. Yamada Takao 山田孝雄. In *NKBT,* vols. 22–26.

Kōyakushō 香薬抄. By Ken'i 兼意. In *ZGR,* vol. 31.1: 57–111.

Kōyōshō 香要抄. By Ken'i 兼意. In 1/ *Jūyō bunkazai* Kōyōshō *(eiin bon)* 1, 2 重要文化財　香要抄（影印本）I, II. 2 vols. Ed. Koizumi Enjun 古泉圓順, Ōsaka 大阪: Takeda Kagaku Shinkō Zaidan 武田科学振興財団, 2008, 2009. 2/ *ZGR*, vol. 31.1: 1–56.

Lingnan weisheng fang 嶺南衛生方. By Jihong 継洪. Zhongyi Guji Chubanshe 中医古籍出版社, 1983.

Mahāparinirvāna Sutra (*Daihatsu nehan gyō* 大般涅槃経). *T.* 12: no. 374. Translated in Kosho Yamamoto, ed. Tony Page, *Mahayana Mahaparinirvana Sutra: The Complete Translation from the Classical Chinese.* London: Nirvana Publications, 2000. Online at http://www.nirvanasutra.org.uk/.

Maka shikan (Ch. *Mohe zhiguan*) 摩訶止観. By Zhiyi 智顗. *T.* 46, no. 1911: 1–140.

Man'anpō 万安方. By Kajiwara Shōzen 梶原性全. Kagaku Shoin 科学書院, 1986.

Minkeiki 民経記. By Hirobashi Tsunemitsu 広橋経光. 10 vols. In *Dai Nihon kokiroku* 大日本古記録. Iwanami Shoten 岩波書店, 1975–2007.

Muchū mondō shū 夢中問答集. By Musō Soseki 夢窓疎石. Ed. and trans. Kawase Kazuma 川瀬一馬. Kōdansha 講談社, 2000.

Nanbokuchō ibun Chūgoku Shikoku hen (*NBI-Ch*) 南北朝遺文中国四国編. Ed. Matsuoka Hisato 松岡久人. 6 vols. Tōkyōdō Shuppan 東京堂出版, 1987–1995.

Nanbokuchō ibun Kantō hen (NBI-Ka) 南北朝遺文関東編. 4 vols. to date. Ed. Satō Kazuhiko 佐藤和彦, Itō Kazuhiko 伊東和彦, Yamada Kuniaki 山田邦明, Tsunoda Tomohiko 角田朋彦, Shimizu Ryō 清水亮. Tokyo: Tōkyōdō Shuppan 東京堂出版, 2007–.

Nanbokuchō ibun Kyūshū hen (*NBI-Ky*) 南北朝遺文九州編. Ed. Seno Seiichirō 瀬野清一郎. 7 vols. Tōkyōdō Shuppan 東京堂出版, 1981–1989.

Nanbokuchō ibun Tōhoku hen (*NBI-To*) 南北朝遺文関東編. Ed. Ōishi Naomasa 大石直正 and Nanami Masato 七海雅人. 1 vol. to date. Tōkyōdō Shuppan 東京堂出版, 2008–.

Nihon koten bungaku taikei (*NKBT*) 日本古典文学大系. 100 vols. Iwanami Shoten 岩波書店, 1958–1968.

Puji benshi fang 普済本事方. By Xu Shuwei 許叔微. Taipei 台北: Xinwenfeng Chuban Gongsi 新文豊出版公司, 1987.

Rencun Sunshi zhibing huofa mifang 仁存孫氏治病活法秘方. By Sun Rencun 孫仁存. Manuscript held in the Naikaku Bunko collection of the National Archives of Japan 国立公文書館内閣文庫所蔵.

Rennyo shōnin ofumi 蓮如上人御文. By Rennyo 蓮如. *T.* 83, no. 2668: 771–808. Translated in: 1/ Minor and Ann Rogers, *Rennyo: The Second Founder of Shin Buddhism, with a Translation of His Letters.* Berkeley: Asian Humanities Press, 1991. 2/ Ann T. Rogers and Minor L. Rogers, *Rennyo Shōnin Ofumi: The Letters of Rennyo.* In *BDK English Tripitaka,* 105-II, 106-I: 9–137. Berkeley: Numata Center for Buddhist Translation and Research, 1996.

Sanyin fang 三因方 (*Sanyin jiyi bingzheng fanglun* 三因極一病証方論). By Chen Yan 陳言. Renmin Weisheng Chubanshe 人民衛生出版社, 1957 (1983 reprint).

Sekiso ōrai 尺素往来. By Ichijō Kaneyoshi 一条兼良. In *GR,* vol. 6: 602–616.

Shaken nichiroku 蔗軒日録. By Shaken 蔗軒. In *Dai Nihon kokiroku* 大日本古記録. Iwanami Shoten 岩波書店, 1953.

Shanghan huorenshu 傷寒活人書. By Zhu Gong 朱肱. In Wang Kentang 王肯堂 comp., *Yitong zhengmai quanshu* 医統正脈全書, as *Zengzhu Shanghan leizheng huorenshu* 增注傷寒類証活人書. Taipei 台北: Xinwenfeng Chuban Gongsi 新文豊出版公司, 1987.

Shanghan lun 傷寒論. By Zhang Zhongjing 張仲景. Translated in Shāng Hán Lùn, *On Cold Damage: Translation and Commentaries.* By Craig Mitchell, Féng Yè, and Nigel Wiseman. Brookline: Paradigm Publications, 1999.

Shasekishū 沙石集 . By Mujū Ichien 無住一円. Ed. Watanabe Tsunaya 渡邊綱也. In *NKBT,* vol. 85. Iwanami Shoten 岩波書店, 1966.

Shenghui fang 聖恵方. See *Taiping Shenghui fang.*

Shengji zonglu 聖済總録. 2 volumes. Renmin Weisheng Chubanshe 人民衛生出版社, 1962 (1982 reprint).

Shinpen Saitama kenshi shiryō hen vol. 5 *chūsei* 1, *komonjo* 1 新編埼玉県史資料編 5.中世 1 古文書 1. Comp. Saitamaken 埼玉県. Urawa 浦和: Saitamaken 埼玉県, 1982.

Shinsarugaku ki 新猿楽記. By Fujiwara Akihira 藤原明衡. In *Kodai seiji shakai shisō* 古代政治社会思想: 134–152. Ed. Yamagishi Tokuhei 山岸徳平 et al. Iwanami Shoten 岩波書店, 1986.

Shizhai baiyi xuanfang 是斎百一選方. By Wang Qiu 王璆. Taipei 台北: Xinwenfeng Chuban Gongsi 新文豊出版公司, 1987.

Shōkenkō 蕉堅藁. By Zekkai Chūshin 絶海中津. In *Gozan bungaku shū* 五山文学集: 1–194. Ed. Iriya Yoshitaka 入矢義高. In *Shin Nihon koten bungaku taikei* 新日本古典文学大系, vol. 48. Iwanami Shoten 岩波書店, 1990.

Shōkō Daitokufu 性公大徳譜. In *Gokuraku Ritsuji shi chūsei kinsei hen* 極楽律寺史中世近世編, qv*:* 73–76.

Taiheiki 太平記. Ed. Gotō Tanji 後藤丹治 and Kamata Kisaburō 釜田喜三郎. 3 vols. In *NKBT,* vols. 34–36. Partial translation in Helen Craig McCullough, *The Taiheiki: A Chronicle of Medieval Japan.* New York: Columbia University Press, 1959.

Taiping huimin Hejiju fang 太平恵民和剤局方. By Chen Shiwen 陳師文 et al. In: 1/ *Kankoku zōkō Taiping Hejiju fang* 官刻増広太平和剤局法. 2 vols. Ryōgen shoten 燎原書店, 1976. 2/ *Kunchū Hejiju fang* 訓注和剤局方. Ed. Yoshitomi Hyōe 吉富兵衛. Yukari Shobō 縁書房, 1992.

Taiping Shenghui fang 太平聖恵方. By Wang Huaiyin 王懐隠. Renmin Weisheng Chubanshe 人民衛生出版社, 1982 reprint.

Taishō shinshū Daizōkyō (T) 大正新脩大蔵経. Ed. Takakusu Junjirō 高楠順次郎 and Watanabe Kaigyoku 渡邊海旭. 85 vols. Taishō Shinshū Daizōkyō Kankōkai 大正新脩大蔵経刊行会, 1924–1935.

Tamon'in nikki 多聞院日記. By Tamon'in Eishun 多聞院英俊. 6 vols. Ed. Tsuji Zennosuke 辻善之助. Kadokawa Shoten 角川書店, 1967.

Tengu zōshi 天狗草紙. In *Zoku Nihon emaki taisei,* 続日本絵巻大成, vol. 19. Ed. Komatsu Shigemi 小松茂実. Chūō Kōron 中央公論, 1984.

Ton'ishō 頓医抄. By Kajiwara Shōzen 梶原性全. 1/ Kagaku Shoin 科学書院, 1986. 2/ Naikaku Bunko 内閣文庫 microfilm hard copy in the collection of the Kitasato Kenkyūjo Tōyō Igaku Sōgō Kenkyūjo Ishigaku Kenkyūbu 北里研究所東洋医学総合研究所医史学研究部所蔵.

Tsūken nyūdō zōsho mokuroku 通憲入道蔵書目録. In *GR,* vol. 21: 545–554.

Waike jingyao 外科精要. By Chen Ziming 陳自明. In Volume 3-2 of the *Wakoku Kanseki isho shūsei* 和刻漢籍医書集成. Ed. Kosoto Hiroshi 小曽戸洋. Entāpuraizu エンタプライズ, 1989.

Weishi jiacang fang 魏氏家蔵方. By Wei Xian 魏峴. 1/ Microfilm copy in the collection of the Kitasato Kenkyūjo Tōyō Igaku Sōgō Kenkyūjo Ishigaku Kenkyūbu 北里研究所東洋医学総合研究所医史学研究部所蔵. 2/ *Beijing Daxue Tushuguan Guancang Shanben Yishu* Weishi jiacang fang 北京大学図書館館蔵善本医書魏氏家蔵方. Zhongguo Guji Yishu Chubanshe 中国古籍医書出版社, 1987.

Writings of Nichiren Daishōnin, The, (WND). Ed. Gosho Translation Committee. Sōka Gakkai, 1999, 2003.

Yakushushō 薬種抄. By Ken'i 兼意. In: 1/ *Jūyō bunkazai* Yakushushō *(eiin bon)* 1, 2 重要文化財　薬種抄（影印本）I, II. 2 vols. Ōsaka 大阪: Takeda Kagaku Shinkō Zaidan 武田科学振興財団, 2010, 2011. 2/ *Tenri toshokan zenpon sōsho Washo no bu* 31 天理図書館善本叢書和書の部31. Yagi Shoten 八木書店, 1977. 3/ *T* (*zuzō* 図像) 11: 177–230.

Yamai no sōshi 病の草紙. In *Gaki zōshi, Jigoku zōshi, Yamai no sōshi, Kuzōshi emaki,* 餓鬼草紙　地獄草紙　病草紙　九相死絵巻. In *Nihon emaki taisei* 日本絵巻大成, vol. 7. Ed. Komatsu Shigemi 小松茂. Chūō Kōronsha 中央公論社, 1977.

Yangshi jiacang fang 楊氏家蔵方. By Yang Tan 楊倓. 2 vols. Taipei 台北: Xinwenfeng Chuban Gongsi 新文豊出版公司, 1987.

Yeshi luyan fang 葉氏録験方. By Ye Dalian 葉大廉. Taipei 台北: Xinwenfeng Chuban Gongsi 新文豊出版公司, 1987.

Youyou xinshu 幼幼新書. By Liu Fang 劉昉 et al. Renmin Weisheng Chubanshe 人民衛生出版社, 1987.

Yuyaoyuan fang 御薬院方. By Xu Guozhen 許国禎. Zhongyi Guji Chubanshe 中医古籍出版社, 1983. 2 vols.

Zenkunen kassen ekotoba 前九年合戦絵詞. In *Zoku Nihon emaki taisei* 続日本絵巻大成, vol. 17. Ed. Komatsu Shigemi 小松茂美. Chūō Kōron Sha 中央公論者, 1983.

Zoku gunsho ruijū (ZGR) 続群書類従. Ed. Hanawa Hokinoichi 塙保己一 and Ōta Tōshirō 大田藤四郎. 34 volumes. Zoku Gunsho Ruijū Kanseikai 続群書類従完成会, 1929–1933.

Secondary Sources

Abé, Ryūichi. "Mantra, Hinin, and the Feminine." *Cahiers d'Extrême-Asie* 13 (2002–2003): 101–125.

Adachihara Akiko 安達原曄子. "*Man'anpō* no shōnimon ni tsuite 万安方の小児門について." *Nihon ishigaku zasshi* 日本医史学雑誌, 29.4 (1983): 353–367.

———. "*Man'anpō* shōnimon ni mirareru *Shanghan lun* no eikyō 万安方小児門にみられる傷寒論の影響." In *Yakazu Dōmei sensei kiju kinen bunshū* 矢数道明先生喜寿記念文集: 281–292. Ed. Onchi Kai 温知会. Onchi Kai 温知会, 1981.

Anthropological Society of Nippon. *Medieval Japanese Skeletons from the Burial Site at Zaimokuza, Kamakura City.* Tokyo: Iwanami Shoten, 1956.

Ariga Yōen 有賀要延. *Kō to bukkyō* 香と仏教. Kokusho Kankōkai 国書刊行会, 1990.

Arntzen, Sonja. *Ikkyū and the Crazy Cloud Anthology.* Tokyo: University of Tokyo Press, 1986.

Asahina Yasuhiko 朝比奈康彦, ed. *Shōsōin no yakubutsu* 正倉院の薬物. Ōsaka 大阪: Shokubutsu Bunken Hakkōkai 植物文献発行会, 1955.

Batten, Bruce. *Gateway to Japan: Hakata in War and Peace, 500–1300.* Honolulu: University of Hawai'i Press, 2006.

———. "An Open and Shut Case? Some Thoughts on Late Heian Overseas Trade." In *Currents in Medieval Japanese History: Essays in Honor of Jeffrey P. Mass:* 303–332. Ed. Gordon M. Berger, Andrew Edmund Goble, Lorraine F. Harrington, and G. Cameron Hurst III. Los Angeles: Figueroa Press, 2009.

Berger, Gordon M., Andrew Edmund Goble, Lorraine F. Harrington, and G. Cameron Hurst III, eds. *Currents in Medieval Japanese History: Essays in Honor of Jeffrey P. Mass.* Los Angeles: Figueroa Press, 2009.

Borgen, Robert. "Jōjin's Discoveries in Song China." In *Tools of Culture: Japan's Cultural, Intellectual, Medical, and Technological Contacts in East Asia, 1000s–1500s:* 25–47. Ed. Andrew Edmund Goble, Kenneth R. Robinson, and Haruko Wakabayashi. Ann Arbor, MI: Association for Asian Studies, 2009.

———. "Jōjin's Travels from Center to Center (with Some Periphery in Between)." In *Heian Japan: Centers and Peripheries:* 384–413. Ed. Mikael Adolphson, Edward Kamens, and Stacie Matsumoto. Honolulu: University of Hawai'i Press, 2006.

Buell, Paul D., and Eugene N. Anderson (appendix by Charles Perry). *A Soup for the Qan: Chinese Dietary Medicine of the Mongol Era as Seen in Hu Szu-Hui's* Yin-shan cheng-yao: *Introduction, Translation, Commentary and Chinese Text.* London and New York: Kegan Paul International, 2000.

Collcutt, Martin. *Five Mountains: The Rinzai Zen Monastic Institution in Medieval Japan.* Cambridge, MA: Council on East Asian Studies, Harvard University, 1981.

———. "Lanxi Daolong (1203–1278) at Kenchōji: Chinese Contributions to the Making of Medieval Japanese Rinzai Zen." In *Tools of Culture: Japan's Cultural, Intellectual, Medical, and Technological Contacts in East Asia, 1000s–1500s:* 135–162. Ed. Andrew Edmund Goble, Kenneth R. Robinson, Haruko Wakabayashi. Ann Arbor, MI: Association for Asian Studies, 2009.

Conlan, Thomas トーマス コンラン. *In Little Need of Divine Intervention: Scrolls of the Mongol Invasions of Japan.* Ithaca: East Asia Program, Cornell University, 2001.

———. "Nambokuchō ki kassen no ichi kōsatsu: sen shishō kara mita tokushitsu 南北朝期合戦の一考察―戦死傷からみた特質." In *Nihon shakai no shiteki kōzō, kodai chūsei* 日本社会の史的構造古代中世: 417–439. Ed. Oyama Kyōhei Kyōjū Taikan Kinenkai 大山喬平教授退官記念会. Kyoto 京都: Shibunkaku Shuppan 思文閣出版, 1997.

———. *State of War: The Violent Order of Fourteenth Century Japan.* Ann Arbor: University of Michigan Center for Japanese Studies, 2003.

Covell, Jon Carter. *Untangling Zen's Red Thread.* New Jersey and Seoul: Hollym International Corporation, 1980.

Dumoulin, Heinrich. *Zen Buddhism: A History.* Vol. 2: *Japan.* New York: Macmillan, 1990.

Farris, William Wayne. *Heavenly Warriors: The Evolution of Japan's Military, 500–1300.* Cambridge, MA: Harvard University Council on East Asian Studies, 1992.

Friday, Karl. *Hired Swords.* Stanford, CA: Stanford University Press, 1992.

———. *Samurai, Warfare and the State in Early Medieval Japan.* London: Routledge, 2004.

———. "What a Difference a Bow Makes: The Rules of War in Early Medieval Japan." In *Currents in Medieval Japanese History: Essays in Honor of Jeffrey P. Mass:* 53–86. Ed. Gordon M. Berger, Andrew Edmund Goble, Lorraine F. Harrington, and G. Cameron Hurst III. Los Angeles: Figueroa Press, 2009.

Fujino Yutaka 藤野豊, ed. *Rekishi no naka no raija* 歴史のなかの癩者. Yumiru Shuppan ゆみる出版, 1996.

Fukunaga Katsumi 福永勝美. *Bukkyō igaku jiten* 仏教医学事典. Yūzankaku Shuppan 雄山閣出版, 1990.

Fukushima Kaneharu 福島金治. *Kanezawa Hōjō shi to Shōmyōji* 金沢北条氏と称名寺. Yoshikawa Kōbunkan 吉川弘文館, 1997.

Furth, Charlotte. *A Flourishing Yin: Gender in China's Medical History, 960–1665.* Berkeley: University of California Press, 1999.

Furuta Shōkin 古田紹欽. *Eisai Kissa yōjō ki* 栄西喫茶養生記. Kōdansha 講談社, 2000.

Goble, Andrew Edmund. "Images of Illness: Interpreting the Medieval *Scrolls of Afflictions.*" In *Currents in Medieval Japanese History: Essays in Honor of Jeffrey P. Mass:* 165–218. Ed. Gordon M. Berger, Andrew Edmund Goble, Lorraine F. Harrington, and G. Cameron Hurst III. Los Angeles: Figueroa Press, 2009.

———. "The Kamakura Bakufu and Its Officials." In *The Bakufu in Japanese History:* 31–48. Ed. Jeffrey P. Mass and William B. Hauser. Stanford, CA: Stanford University Press, 1985.

———. *Kenmu: Go-Daigo's Revolution.* Cambridge, MA: Harvard University Council on East Asian Studies, 1996.

———. "Nichiren Calming Karma: Sickness, Fear, and Lotus unto Death." In *Deep Hearing in Buddhism and Psychotherapy.* Ed. Richard K. Payne and Mark T. Unno (forthcoming, Wisdom Publications).

———. "War and Injury: The Emergence of Wound Medicine in Medieval Japan." *Monumenta Nipponica* 60.3 (autumn 2005): 297–338.

Goble, Andrew Edmund, Kenneth R. Robinson, and Haruko Wakabayashi. "Introduction: The Ubiquity of Contacts." In *Tools of Culture: Japan's Cultural, Intellectual, Medical, and Technological Contacts in East Asia, 1000s–1500s:* 1–21. Ed. Andrew Edmund Goble, Kenneth R. Robinson, and Haruko Wakabayashi. Ann Arbor, MI: Association for Asian Studies, 2009.

———, eds. *Tools of Culture: Japan's Cultural, Intellectual, Medical, and Technological Contacts in East Asia, 1000s–1500s.* Ann Arbor, MI: Association for Asian Studies, 2009.

Goodwin, Janet R. *Alms and Vagabonds: Buddhist Temples and Popular Patronage in Medieval Japan.* Honolulu: University of Hawai'i Press, 1994.

Gosho Translation Committee. *The Writings of Nichiren Daishōnin.* Tōkyō: Sōka Gakkai, 1999, 2003. Also online at http://sgi-usa.org/Buddhism/library/Nichiren/wnd.

Gu Wembi 顧文璧 and Lin Shimin 林士民. "Neiha [Ningbo] ni genzon suru Nihon koku Dazaifu Hakata tsu no kakyō kokuseki no kenkyū 寧波に現存する日本国大宰府博多津の華僑刻石の研究." *Kaijishi kenkyū* 海事史研究 43 (1986.6): 101–112.

Guo Xiumei 郭秀梅 and Kosoto Hiroshi 小曽戸洋. *Man'anpō in'yō shomei sakuin* 万安方引用書名索引. Unpublished manuscript, 1998.

Guo Xiumei 郭秀梅, Kosoto Hiroshi 小曽戸洋, and Okada Kenkichi 岡田研吉. "*Man'anpō* yin Zhongguo yishu guankai 万安方引中国医書管窺." *Journal of Chinese Medicine* 9.3 (1998): 127–135.

Hattori Toshirō 服部敏郎. *Heian jidai igakushi no kenkyū* 平安時代医学史の研究. Yoshikawa Kōbunkan 吉川弘文館, 1955.

———. *Igaku* 医学. Kondō Shuppansha 近藤出版社, 1985.

———. *Kamakura jidai igakushi no kenkyū* 鎌倉時代医学史の研究. Yoshikawa Kōbunkan 吉川弘文館, 1964.

———. *Muromachi Azuchi Momoyama jidai igakushi no kenkyū* 室町安土桃山時代医学史の研究. Yoshikawa Kōbunkan 吉川弘文館, 1971.

———. *Nara jidai igakushi no kenkyū* 奈良時代医学史の研究. Yoshikawa Kōbunkan 吉川弘文館, 1988 (orig. published 1945).

Hayakawa Shōhachi 早川庄八. *Shoku Nihongi* 続日本紀. Iwanami Shoten 岩波書店, 1993.

Higuchi Seitarō 樋口誠太郎. "*Azuma kagami* o chūshin toshite mita Kamakura ishi 吾妻鏡を中心としてみた鎌倉医師." *Nihon ishigaku zasshi* 日本医史学雑誌 18 (1972): 246–257.

Hirata Kazuaki 平田和明. "Kamakura shutsudo jinkotsu no kotsubyōhen－Yuigahama minami iseki shutsudo jinkotsu o chūshin ni 鎌倉出土人骨の骨病変－由比ケ浜南遺跡出土人骨を中心に." In *Chūsei toshi Kamakura to shi no sekai* 中世都市鎌倉と死の世界: 29–45. Ed. Gomi Fumihiko 五味文彦 and Saiki Hideo 斎木秀雄. Takashi Shoin 高志書院, 2002.

Hosokawa Ryōichi 細川涼一. *Kanjin gakushōki – Saidaiji Eison no jiden* 感身学正記－西大寺叡尊の自伝. Heibonsha 平凡社, 1999.

———. "Ninshō no shōgai 忍性の生涯." In *Eison, Ninshō* 叡尊, 忍性: 111–141. Ed. Matsuo Kenji 松尾剛次. Yoshikawa Kōbunkan 吉川弘文館, 2004.

Hosokawa Shigeo 細川重男. "Mandokoro shitsuji Nikaidō shi ni tsuite 政所執事二階堂氏について." In *Kamakura jidai no shakai to bunka* 鎌倉時代の社会と文化: 215–251. Ed. Kamakura Ibun Kenkyūkai 鎌倉遺文研究会. Yoshikawa Kōbunkan 吉川弘文館, 1999.

Hsia, Emil, Ilza Veith, and Robert Geertsma, trans. *The Essentials of Medicine in Ancient China and Japan: Yasuyori Tanba's Ishinpō.* Leiden: Brill, 1986.

Hu, Shiu-ying. *An Enumeration of Chinese Materia Medica.* 2nd. ed. Ann Arbor: University of Michigan Press, 1999.

Ishihara Akira 石原明. "*Eisei hiyōshō* 衛生秘要抄." In *Gunsho kaidai* 群書解題, vol. 5: 288. Ed. Zoku Gunsho Ruijū Kanseikai 続群書類従完成会. Zoku Gunsho Ruijū Kanseikai 続群書類従完成会, 1960.

———. "*Honzō iroha shō* kaidai 本草色葉鈔解題." In *Honzō iroha shō* 本草色葉鈔. Ed. Ishihara Akira 石原明. Naikaku Bunko 内閣文庫, 1968.

———. "Kajiwara Shōzen no shōgai to sono chosho 梶原性全の生涯とその著書." In *Man'anpō* (Kagaku Shoin 科学書院, 1986): 1731–1752. The original essay appears in *Nihon ishigaku zasshi* 日本医史学雑誌, 6.2 (1956): 9–20, and 6.4 (1956): 7–28.

Ishii Susumu 石井進. "Toshi Kamakura ni okeru 'jigoku' no fūkei 都市鎌倉における「地獄」の風景." In *Shōensei to buke shakai* 荘園制と武家社会: 77–112. Ed. Gokeninsei Kenkyūkai 御家人制研究会. Yoshikawa Kōbunkan 吉川弘文館, 1981.

Iwama Machiko 岩間眞知子. *Cha no iyakushi* 茶の医薬史. Kyoto 京都: Shibunkaku Shuppan 思文閣出版, 2009.

Johnston, William. *The Modern Epidemic: A History of Tuberculosis in Japan.* Cambridge, MA: Council on East Asian Studies, 1995.

Kakehi Masahiro 筧雅博. *Mōko shūrai to tokusei rei* 蒙古襲来と徳政令. Kōdansha 講談社, 2009.

Kanagawa Kenritsu Kanazawa Bunko 神奈川県立金沢文庫, ed. *Cha to Kanezawa Sadaaki* 茶と金沢貞顕. Yokohama 横浜: Kanagawa Kenritsu Kanazawa Bunko 神奈川県立金沢文庫, 2005.

———. *Karamono to Sōban Issaikyō* 唐物と宋版一切経. Yokohama 横浜: Kanagawa Kenritsu Kanazawa Bunko 神奈川県立金沢文庫, 1998.

Kanai Kiyomitsu 金井清光. *Chūsei no raija to sabetsu* 中世の癩者と差別. Iwata Shoin 岩田書院, 2003.

Karasulas, Anthony. "Zaimokuza Reconsidered: The Forensic Evidence, and Classical Japanese Swordsmanship." *World Archaeology* 36.4 (December 2004): 507–518.

Kawazoe Shōji 川添昭二. "Jōtenji no kaisō to Hakata gōshu Sha Kokumei: Kamakura chūki no taigai kankei to Hakata 承天寺の開創と博多綱首謝国明ー鎌倉中期の対外関係と博多." In *Hakata Jōtenji shi, hoi* 博多承天寺史補遺: 1–41. Ed. Hirowata Masatoshi 広渡正利. Hakata 博多: Jōtenji 承天寺, 1990.

Kitagawa Hiroshi and Bruce Tsuchida. *The Tale of the Heike.* University of Tokyo Press, 1975.

Kobayashi Shigefumi 小林茂文. "Kodai chūsei raija to shūkyō 古代中世癩者と宗教." In *Rekishi no naka no raija* 歴史のなかの癩者: 13–79. Ed. Fujino Yutaka 藤野豊. Yumiru Shuppan ゆみる出版, 1996.

Koizumi Enjun 古泉圓順. "Mikkyō to honzō 密教と本草." *Kyōu* 杏雨 1 (*sōkan* 創刊, 1998): 21–54.

Koizumi Yoshiaki 小泉宜右. "Gokenin Nagai shi ni tsuite 御家人長井氏について." In *Takahashi Ryūzō sensei kiju kinen ronshū Kokiroku no kenkyū* 高橋隆三先生喜寿記念論集古記録の研究: 707–765. Ed. Takahashi Ryūzō sensei kiju kinen kai 高橋隆三先生喜寿記念会. Yoshikawa Kōbunkan 吉川弘文館, 1970.

Kojima Takayuki 小島孝之. "Mujū denki shokō－ijutsu to shisō wo megutte 無住伝記小考－医術と思想をめぐって." *Kokugo to kokubungaku* 国語と国文学 1975.12 (52.12): 41–54.

Kosoto Hiroshi 小曽戸洋. *Chūgoku igaku koten to Nihon* 中国医学古典と日本. Hanawa Shobō 塙書房, 1996.

———. "Gendai no iyakusho (1)–(6) 元代の医薬書." *Gendai Tōyō igaku* 現代東洋医学 (1) 11.3 (1990.7): 92–96; (2) 11.4 (1990.10): 76–82; (3) 12.1 (1991.1): 78–85; (4) 12.2 (1991.4): 93–99; (5) 12.3 (1991.7): 94–101; (6) 12.4 (1991.10): 103–109.

———. "Hokusō jidai no iyakusho (sono 1) 北宋時代の医薬書その１." *Gendai Tōyō igaku* 現代東洋医学 8.3 (1987.7): 83–91; and (sono 2) 8.4 (1987.10): 86–95.

———. "*Ishinpō* in'yō bunkenmei sakuin 医心方引用文献名索引." *Nihon ishigaku zasshi* 日本医史学雑誌 32.1 (1986.1): 89–118 (part 1); and 32.3 (1986.7): 333–352 (part 2).

———. "Kansu bon kara Sōgenban e－chūsei Nihon ni okeru Chūgoku isho juyō no yōsō 巻子本から宋元版へ－中世日本における中国医書受容の様相." *Nihon ishigaku zasshi* 日本医史学雑誌 44.4 (1998.12): 451–480.

———. "Kindai no iyakusho (1)–(4) 金代の医薬書." *Gendai Tōyō igaku* 現代東洋医学 (1) 10.3 (1989.7): 101–107; (2) 10.4 (1989.10): 105–112; (3) 11.1 (1990.1): 108–113; (4) 11.2 (1990.4): 99–105.

———. "Koisho dankan *Shinpukuji shozō reihon Kanzōgan tō hō* kō 古医書断簡真福寺所蔵零本甘草丸等方考." In *Yakazu Dōmei sensei tainin kinen Tōyō igaku ronshū* 矢数道明先生退任記念東洋医学論集: 179–189. Ed. Ōtsuka

Yasuo 大塚恭男, Chŏng Chongchŏl 丁宗鉄, Kosoto Hiroshi 小曽戸洋, and Kunida Kinji 国田欣二. Kitasato Kenkyūjo Fuzoku Tōyō Igaku Sōgō Kenkyūjo 北里研究所付属東洋医学総合研究所, 1986.

———. "Nansō jidai no iyakusho (1)–(6) 南宋時代の医薬書." *Gendai Tōyō igaku* 現代東洋医学 (1) 9.1 (1988.1): 87–93; (2) 9.2 (1988.4): 79–85; (3) 9.3 (1988.7): 96–104; (4) 9.4 (1988.10): 96–103; (5) 10.1 (1989.1): 93–99; (6) 10.2 (1989.4): 94–103.

———. *Nihon kanpō tenseki jiten* 日本漢方典籍辞典. Taishūkan Shoten 大修館書店, 1999.

———. "*Taiping huimin Hejiju fang* kaidai 2 太平恵民和剤局方解題 2." In *Zōkō Taiping huimin Hejiju fang* 増広太平恵民和剤局方 (*Wakoku kanseki isho shūsei* 和刻漢籍医書集成 vol. 4). Ed. Kosoto Hiroshi 小曽戸洋 and Mayanagi Makoto 真柳誠. Entapuraizu エンタプライズ, 1988.

———. "Volumes of Knowledge: Observations on Song-Period Printed Medical Texts." In *Tools of Culture: Japan's Cultural, Intellectual, Medical, and Technological Interactions in East Asia, 1000s–1500s:* 211–230. Ed. Andrew Edmund Goble, Kenneth R. Robinson, Haruko Wakabayashi. Ann Arbor, MI: Association for Asian Studies, 2009.

Kuroda Hideo 黒田日出男. *Kyōkai no chūsei, shōchō no chūsei* 境界の中世象徴の中世. Tōkyō Daigaku Shuppankai 東京大学出版会, 1986.

Kyōtofu Ishikai, ed. 京都府医史会編. *Kyōto no igakushi* 京都の医学史. Kyōto 京都: Shibunkaku Shuppan 思文閣出版, 1975.

LaFleur, William. "Hungry Ghosts and Hungry People: Somaticity and Rationality in Medieval Japan." In *Fragments for a History of the Human Body, Part One:* 270–303. Ed. Michel Feher. New York: Zone Publications, 1989.

Levy, Howard, and Ishihara Akira, trans. *The Tao of Sex: An Annotated Translation of the Twenty-Eighth Section of the Essence of Medical Prescriptions (Ishinpō).* Yokohama: Shibundō, 1968.

Liu Shukui 劉書奎. "*Youyou xinshu* yinyong yixue wenxian kao 幼幼新書引用医学文献考." *Zhonghua yishi zazhi* 中華医史雑誌 28.3 (1998): 177–180.

Mabuchi Kazuo 馬淵和雄. *Kamakura Daibutsu no chūseishi* 鎌倉大仏の中世史. Shin Jinbutsu Ōraisha 新人物大来社, 1998.

Maejima Norimoto 前島己基. "Nihon kodai no kōhaku no michi 日本古代の琥珀の道." *Museum* 443 (1988): 4–9.

Mass, Jeffrey P. "Of Hierarchy and Authority at the End of Kamakura." In *The Origins of Japan's Medieval World:* 17–38. Ed. Jeffrey P. Mass. Stanford, CA: Stanford University Press, 1997.

———. *Yoritomo and the Founding of the First Bakufu: The Origins of Dual Government in Japan.* Stanford, CA: Stanford University Press, 1999.

Matisoff, Susan. "Holy Horrors: The Sermon Ballads of Medieval and Early Modern Japan." In *Flowing Traces: Buddhism in the Literary and Visual Arts of Japan:* 234–261. Ed. James H. Sanford, William R. LaFleur, and Masatoshi Nagatomi. Princeton, NJ: Princeton University Press, 1992.

Matsuo Kenji 松尾剛次. *Chūsei no toshi to hinin* 中世の都市と非人. Kyōto 京都: Hōzōkan 宝蔵館, 1998.

———, ed. *Eison, Ninshō* 叡尊, 忍性. Yoshikawa Kōbunkan 吉川弘文館, 2004.

———. "Hakata Daijōji to chūsei toshi Hakata 博多大乗寺と中世都市博多." *Kamakura ibun kenkyū* 鎌倉遺文研究 18 (2006.10): 26–39.

———. *Ninshō* 忍性. Minerubua Shobō ミネルヴァ書房, 2004.

Mayanagi Makoto 真柳誠. "*Honzō iroha shō* shoin no igaku bunken 本草色葉鈔書引の医学文献." *Nihon ishigaku zasshi* 日本医史学雑誌 36.1 (1990.3): 34–36.

———. "*Honzō wamyō* in'yō shomei sakuin 本草和名引用書名索引." *Nihon ishigaku zasshi* 日本医史学雑誌 33.3 (1987): 381–396.

———. "*Jingui yaolüe* no seiritsu to genzon hanpon 金匱要略の成立と現存版本." *Kanpō no rinshō* 漢方の臨床 57.3 (2010): 405–420.

McCullough, Helen Craig, trans. *The Taiheiki: A Chronicle of Medieval Japan.* New York: Columbia University Press, 1959.

———. "A Tale of Mutsu." *Harvard Journal of Asiatic Studies* 25 (1964–1965): 178–211.

———, trans. *The Tale of the Heike.* Stanford, CA: Stanford University Press, 1988.

McCullough, William H. "The *Azuma Kagami* Account of the Shōkyū War." *Monumenta Nipponica* 23.1/2 (1968): 102–155.

Meeks, Lori. *Hokkeji and the Reemergence of Female Monasticism in Medieval Japan.* Honolulu: University of Hawai'i Press, 2010.

Moon, Hyungsub. "The Matsura Pirate-Warriors of Northwestern Kyushu in the Kamakura Age." In *Currents in Medieval Japanese History: Essays in Honor of Jeffrey P. Mass:* 363–399. Ed. Gordon M. Berger, Andrew Edmund Goble, Lorraine F. Harrington, and G. Cameron Hurst III. Los Angeles: Figueroa Press, 2009.

Mori Shikazō 森鹿三. *Honzōgaku kenkyū* 本草学研究. Ōsaka 大阪: Kyōu Shooku 杏雨書屋, 1999.

———. "Shōsōin yakubutsu to shuju yakuchō 正倉院薬物と種々薬帳." In Asahina Yasuhiko ed., *Shōsōin no yakubutsu,* qv: 17–67.

Morrell, Robert. *Sand and Pebbles (Shasekishū).* Albany: State University of New York Press, 1985.

Murai Shōsuke 村井章介. *Nanbokuchō no dōran* 南北朝の動乱. Yoshikawa Kōbunkan 吉川弘文館, 2003.

Nagai Chū 長井忠. "*Ishinpō* o chūshin to seru Nihon kodai no gunjin geka 医心方を中心とせる日本古代の軍人外科." *Nihon ishigaku zasshi* 日本医史学雑誌 1324 (1944): 47–55.

Nagai Susumu 長井晋. *Kanezawa Hōjō shi no kenkyū* 金沢北条氏の研究. Yagi Shoten 八木書店, 2006.

———. *Kanezawa Sadaaki* 金沢貞顕. Yoshikawa Kōbunkan 吉川弘文館, 2003.

Nakajima Gakushō 中島楽章. "Eiraku nenkan no Nichimin chōkō bōeki 永楽年間の日明朝貢貿易." *Shien* 史淵 140 (2003.3): 51–99.

Nakamura Ken 中村研. "Jitō hihō to katakana gonjōjō 地頭非法と片仮名言上状." In *Shōen no sekai* 荘園の世界: 203–237. Ed. Inagaki Yasuhiko 稲垣泰彦. Tōkyō Daigaku Shuppankai 東京大学出版会, 1973.

Nakamura Teruko 中村輝子, Kawaguchi Naomi 川口直美, and Endō Jirō 遠藤次郎. "*Hejiju fang* shōkanhen no kentō 和剤局方傷寒篇の検討." *Yakushigaku zasshi* 薬史学雑誌 35.2 (2000): 218–223.

Nakamura Teruko 中村輝子, Matsuzaki Aiko 松崎亜衣子, and Endō Jirō 遠藤次郎. "*Hejiju fang* issaikihen no kentō 和剤局方一切気篇の検討." *Kanpō no rinshō* 漢方の臨床 47.11 (2000.11): 119–126.

———. "*Hejiju fang* ni okeru hōkōsei ken'i yaku no kentō－seiiki no igaku no eikyō ni tsuite 和剤局方における芳香性健胃薬の検討－西域の医学の影響について." *Yakushigaku zasshi* 薬史学雑誌 35.2 (2000): 153–158.

Nakamura Teruko 中村輝子, Miyamoto Hirokazu 宮本浩和, and Endō Jirō 遠藤次郎. "*Hejiju fang* ni mirareru seizai no tokuchō 和剤局方に見られる製剤の特徴." *Yakushigaku zasshi* 薬史学雑誌 38.2 (2003): 185–192.

Nelson, Thomas. "Slavery in Medieval Japan." *Monumenta Nipponica* 59.4 (winter 2004): 463–492.

Nishioka Reizō 西岡禮三 and Yanagita Yoshitaka 柳田純孝. *Genkō to Hakata: Shashin de yomu Mōko shūrai* 元寇と博多ー写真で読む蒙古襲来. Fukuoka 福岡: Nishi Nihon Shinbunsha 西日本新聞社, 2001.

Nojiri Tadashi 野尻忠. "Kinryō kisai kara mita Shōsōin tan uramonjo no kenkyū 斤量記載からみた正倉院丹裏文書の研究." *Komonjo kenkyū* 古文書研究 57 (2003.5): 1–29.

Okanishi Tameto 岡西為人. "Chūgoku honzō no torai to sono eikyō 中国本草の渡来と其影響." In *Meijizen Nihon yakubutsugakushi* 明治前日本薬物学史, vol. 2: 1–265. Ed. Nihon Gakushiin 日本学士院. Zaidan Hōjin Nihon Koigaku Shiryō Sentā 財団法人日本古医学資料センター, 1978.

———. *Honzō gaisetsu* 本草概説. Ōsaka 大阪: Sōgensha 創元社, 1977.

Okazaki Kanzō 岡崎寛蔵. *Kusuri no rekishi* くすりの歴史. Kōdansha 講談社, 1976.

Ōsumi Kazuo 大隅和雄. *Shinshin no sekai, tonseisha no kokoro* 信心の世界、遁世者の心. Chūō Kōronsha 中央公論社者, 2002.

Ōtsuka Norihiro 大塚紀弘. "Sōban *Issaikyō* no yu'nyū to juyō 宋版一切経の輸入と受容." *Kamakura ibun kenkyū* 鎌倉遺文研究 25 (2010.4), 42–70.

Pollack, David. *Zen Poems of the Five Mountains.* New York: Crossroad Publishing Company; Decatur: Scholars Press, 1985.

Quinter, David Ralph. "Creating Bodhisattvas: Eison, *Hinin,* and the 'Living Mañjuśrī.'" *Monumenta Nipponica* 62.4 (winter 2007): 437–479.

———. "The Shingon Ritsu School and the Mañjuśrī Cult in the Kamakura Period: From Eison to Monkan." Doctoral Dissertation, Stanford University, 2006.

Reischauer, Edwin O., trans. *Ennin's Diary: The Record of a Pilgrimage to China in Search of the Law.* New York: Ronald Press, 1955.

———. *Ennin's Travels in T'ang China.* New York: Ronald Press, 1955.

Rogers, Ann, and Minor Rogers. *Rennyo: The Second Founder of Shin Buddhism, with a Translation of His Letters.* Berkeley, CA: Asian Humanities Press, 1991.

Rossabi, Morris. *Khubilai Khan: His Life and Times.* Berkeley: University of California Press, 1988.

Saeki, Kōji 佐伯弘次. "Chinese Trade Ceramics in Medieval Japan." In *Tools of Culture: Japan's Cultural, Intellectual, Medical, and Technological Contacts in East Asia, 1000s–1500s:* 163–182. Ed. Andrew Edmund Goble, Kenneth R. Robinson, Haruko Wakabayashi. Ann Arbor, MI: Association for Asian Studies, 2009.

———. *Mongoru shūrai no totsugeki* モンゴル襲来の衝撃. Chūō Kōron Shinsha 中央公論新社, 2003.

Sakai Shizu 酒井シヅ. *Nihon no iryōshi* 日本の医療史. Tokyo Shoseki Kabushiki Kaisha 東京書籍株式会社, 1982.

Sanson, Sir George. *A History of Japan, 1334 to 1615.* Stanford, CA: Stanford University Press, 1959.

———. *A History of Japan to 1334.* Stanford, CA: Stanford University Press, 1958.

Sasaki Kaoru 佐々木馨. *Nichiren to sono shisō* 日蓮とその思想. Kyōto 京都: Heirakuji Shoten 平楽時書店, 2004.

Sasaki Toshikazu 佐々木利和. "Hakubutsukan shomoku shikō Teishitsu bon no bu Igakukan hon hen, Yūrin *Fukudenpō* ni tsuite 博物館書目誌稿帝室本之部医学館本編有林福田方について." *Museum* 518 (1994.5): 4–13 (part 1), and 538 (1995.8): 30–34 (part 2).

Segal, Ethan. "Awash with Coins: The Spread of Money in Medieval Japan." In *Currents in Medieval Japanese History: Essays in Honor of Jeffrey P. Mass:* 331–361. Ed. Gordon M. Berger, Andrew Edmund Goble, Lorraine F. Harrington, and G. Cameron Hurst III. Los Angeles: Figueroa Press, 2009.

Seki Shūichi 関周一. "Kōryō no michi to Nihon, Chōsen 香料の道と日本朝鮮." In *Ajia no naka no Nihonshi, III, kaijō no michi* アジアのなかの日本史, III, 海上の道: 265–280. Ed. Arano Yasunori 荒野泰典, Ishii Masatoshi 石井正敏, and Murai Shōsuke 村井章介. Tōkyō Daigaku Shuppankai 東京大学出版会, 1992.

Seki Yasushi 関靖. "Hōjō Sanetoki 北条実時." In *Hōjō Yasutoki, Hōjō Sanetoki* 北条泰時, 北条実時: 1–108. Nakamura Hikaru 中村光 and Seki Yasushi 関靖. Hokkai Shuppansha 北海出版社, 1937.

———. *Kanazawa bunko no kenkyū* 金沢文庫の研究. Ōzorasha 大空社, 1992 (reprint).

Sekiguchi Shindai 関口真大, ed. *Maka shikan: Zen no shisō genri* 摩訶止観: 禅の思想原理. Iwanami Shoten 岩波書店, 1966.

Seno Seiichirō 瀬野精一郎. "Kamakura ni okeru totōsen no sōnan ni miru tokusō ke bōeki dokusen no ichi keitai 鎌倉に於ける渡唐船の遭難に見る得宗家貿易独占の一形態." In *Nihon komonjo gaku ronshū 5, Chūsei 1* 日本古文書学論集 5 中世 1: 372–383. Ed. Seno Seiichirō 瀬野精一郎 and Murai Shōsuke 村井章介. Tokyo: Yoshikawa Kōbunkan 吉川弘文館, 1988.

Shackley, Myra. "Arms and the Men: 14th Century Japanese Swordsmanship Illustrated by Skeletons from Zaimokuza, Near Kamakura, Japan." *World Archaeology* 18.2 (October 1986): 247–254.

Shakadō Mitsuhiro 釈迦堂光浩. "Nanbokuchō ki kassen ni okeru senjō 南北朝期合戦における戦傷." *Chūsei nairanshi kenkyū* 中世内乱史研究 13 (1992): 27–39.

Shibata Shōji 柴田承二, ed. *Hōryūji shozō Iyaku chōzai koshō* 法隆寺所蔵医薬調剤古抄. Hirokawa Shoten 廣川書店, 1997.

Shinmura Taku 新村拓. *Kodai iryō kanjinsei no kenkyū* 古代医療官人制の研究. Hōsei Daigaku Shuppan Kyoku 法政大学出版局, 1983.

———. *Nihon iryō shakaishi no kenkyū* 日本医療社会史の研究. Hōsei Daigaku Shuppan Kyoku 法政大学出版局, 1985.

———. "Yamai no zuzō hyōgen 病の図像表現." In *Ippen hijirie o yomitōku* 一遍聖絵を読み解く: 162–180. Ed. Takeda Sachiko 武田佐知子. Yoshikawa Kōbunkan 吉川弘文館, 1999.

Shinoda, Minoru. *The Founding of the Kamakura Shogunate, 1180–1185:* With Selected Translations from the *Azuma Kagami.* New York: Columbia University Press, 1960.

Shiraishi Kogetsu 白石虎月, ed. *Tōfukuji shi* 東福寺誌. Kyōto 京都: Shibunkaku Shuppan 思文閣出版, 1979.

Sivin, Nathan. "Emotional Counter-Therapy." In Nathan Sivin, *Medicine, Religion and Philosophy in Ancient China: Researches and Reflections,* chapter 2: 1–19. Aldershot, UK: Variorum, 1995.

Skord, Virginia. *Tales of Tears and Laughter.* Honolulu: University of Hawai'i Press, 1991.

Smits, Ivo. "China as Classic Text: Chinese Books and Twelfth Century Japanese Collectors." In *Tools of Culture: Japan's Cultural, Intellectual, Medical, and Technological Contacts in East Asia, 1000s–1500s:* 185–210. Ed. Andrew Edmund Goble, Kenneth R. Robinson, and Haruko Wakabayashi. Ann Arbor, MI: Association for Asian Studies, 2009.

Sōda Bunko Mokuroku Henshū Iinkai 宗田文庫目録編集委員会, ed. *Sōda Bunko Mokuroku shoseki hen* 宗田文庫目録書籍篇. Kyōto 京都: Kokusai Nihon Bunka Kenkyū Sentā 国際日本文化研究センター, 2001.

Steenstrup, Carl. *Hōjō Shigetoki (1198–1261) and His Role in the History of Political and Ethical Ideas in Japan.* Scandinavian Institute of Asian Studies monograph. London and Malmo: Curzon Press, 1979.

Sugimoto, Masayoshi, and David L. Swain. *Science and Culture in Traditional Japan, A.D. 600–1854.* Cambridge, MA: MIT Press, 1978.

Sugitatsu Yoshikazu 杉立義一, ed. *Ishinpō no denrai* 医心方の伝来. Kyoto 京都: Shibunkaku Shuppan 思文閣出版, 1991.

Sunagawa Hiroshi 砂川博. "Ishō toshite no Ippen" 医聖としての一遍. In *Ippen Hijiri-e no sōgō teki kenkyū* 一遍聖絵の総合的研究: 171–181. Ed. Sunagawa Hiroshi 砂川博. Iwata Shoin 岩田書院, 2002.

Suzuki Noriko 鈴木則子. "Shodai Manase Dōsan no rai igaku 初代曲直瀬道三の癩医学." *Nihon ishigaku zasshi* 日本医史学雑誌 41.3 (1995): 349–368.

Suzuki Tatsuhiko 鈴木達彦. "*Hejiju fang* no Shōkō, Hōkei, Jun'yū jidai no hensan hōhō to ito 和剤局方の紹興，宝慶，淳祐時代の編纂方法と意図." *Yakushigaku zasshi* 薬史学雑誌 43.1 (2008): 5–12.

———. "*Hejiju fang* no zōho nendai no mondai 和剤局方の増補年代の問題." *Nihon ishigaku zasshi* 日本医史学雑誌 54.1 (2008): 31–38.

Takahashi Shintarō 高橋真太郎. "Chūgoku no yakubutsu ryōhō to sono eikyō 中国の薬物療法と其影響." In *Meijizen Nihon yakubutsugakushi* 明治前日本薬物学史, vol. 2: 267–513. Ed. Nihon Gakushiin 日本学士院. Zaidan Hōjin Nihon Koigaku Shiryō Sentā 財団法人日本古医学資料センター, 1978.

Tanaka Fumihide 田中文英. "Chūsei kenmitsu jiin ni okeru shūhō no ichi kōsatsu 中世顕密寺院における修法の一考察." In *Chūsei jiinshi no kenkyū* 中世寺院史の研究, 1: 161–183. Ed. Chūsei Jiinshi Kenkyūkai 中世寺院史研究会. Kyōto 京都: Hōzōkan 宝蔵館, 1988.

Tōno Haruyuki 東野治之. *Kentōshi to Shōsōin* 遣唐使と正倉院. Iwanami Shoten 岩波書店, 1992.

Ts'ao, Yung-ho. "Pepper Trade in East Asia." *T'oung Pao,* 68.4-5 (1982): 221–247.

Ueda Jun'ichi 上田純一. "Tōfukuji to Saidaiji－jibyō Monjū shinkō wo megutte 東福寺と西大寺－持病文殊信仰をめぐって." *Nihon rekishi* 日本歴史 537 (1993): 18–34.

Ulak, James. "*Fukutomi zōshi:* The Genesis and Transmutations of a Medieval Japanese Scatological Tale." Ph.D. dissertation, Case Western Reserve University, 1994.

Urushibara Tōru 漆原徹. *Chūsei gunchūjō to sono sekai* 中世軍中状とその世界. Yoshikawa Kōbunkan 吉川弘文館, 1998.

Varley, H. Paul. *Warriors of Japan as Portrayed in the War Tales.* Honolulu: University of Hawai'i Press, 1994.

Verschuer, Charlotte von. *Across the Perilous Seas: Japanese Trade with China and Korea from the Seventh to Sixteenth Centuries.* Trans. Kristen Lee Hunter. Ithaca, NY: East Asia Program, Cornell University, 2006.

Wajima Yoshio 和島芳男. *Eison, Ninshō* 叡尊,忍性. Yoshikawa Kōbunkan 吉川弘文館, 1959.

Watanabe Kōzō 渡辺幸三. *Honzōsho no kenkyū* 本草書の研究. Osaka 大阪: Takeda Kagaku Shinkō Zaidan 武田科学振興財団, 1987.

Watanabe Takeshi 渡辺武, Komai Hiroyuki 古米弘幸, and Nakajima Kōji 中島鉱二. "Ganjin ōshō no hihō Karirokugan no saiken to *Ishinpō* fūbyō hen, gendai-yaku no goyaku 鑑真大和上の秘方訶梨漉勒丸の再現と医心方風病篇現代訳の誤訳." *Kanpō no rinshō* 漢方の臨床 35.6 (1988): 45–58.

Watson, Burton, trans. *Han Fei Tzu: Basic Writings.* New York: Columbia University Press, 1964.

———, trans. *The Lotus Sutra.* New York: Columbia University Press, 1983.

Wilms, Sabine. "'Ten Times More Difficult to Treat': Female Bodies in Medical Texts from Early Imperial China." In *Medicine for Women In Imperial China:* 74–107. Ed. Angela Ki Che Leung. Leiden: Brill, 2006.

Wilson, William. *Hōgen Monogatari: Tale of the Disorder in Hōgen.* Tokyo: Voyager's Press (for Monumenta Nipponica), 1971.

Yamada Shigemasa 山田重正. "Kajiwara Shōzen to sono shūi 梶原性全とその周囲." *Hanazono daigaku kenkyū kiyō* 花園大学研究紀要 1 (*sōsetsu gō* 創設号, 1970): 309–341.

———. *Ten'i no rekishi* 典医の歴史. Kyoto 京都: Shibunkaku Shuppan 思文閣出版, 1980.

Yanagihara Toshiaki 柳原俊昭. "Chūsei zenki minami Kyūshū no minato to Sōjin kyoryūchi ni kansuru ichi shiron 中世前紀南九州の港と宋人居留地に関する一試論." *Nihonshi kenkyū* 日本史研究 448 (1999.12): 102–134.

Yokota Noriko 横田則子. "*Monoyoshi* kō: kinsei Kyoto no raija ni tsuite 物吉考－近世京都の癩者に就いて." *Nihonshi kenkyū* 日本史研究 352 (1991): 1–29.

Yoshida Fumio 吉田文夫. "Ninshō no shakai jigyō ni tsuite 忍性の社会事業について." In *Chōgen, Eison, Ninshō* 重源, 叡尊, 忍性: 392–433. Ed. Nakao Takashi 中尾堯 and Imai Masaharu 今井雅晴. Yoshikawa Kōbunkan 吉川弘文館, 1983.

———. "Saidaiji Eison no Kantō gekō 西大寺叡尊の関東下向." In *Chōgen, Eison, Ninshō* 重源, 叡尊, 忍性: 221–248. Ed. Nakao Takashi 中尾堯 and Imai Masaharu 今井雅晴. Yoshikawa Kōbunkan 吉川弘文館, 1983.

Zysk, Kenneth. *Asceticism and Healing in Ancient India.* New York: Oxford University Press, 1991.

INDEX

agada medicine, 65, 99, 142 n. 77
"all forms of [disorders of] qi," 57, 58, 59, 60, 62, 63, 64, 102, 141 n. 60; first articulated in *Hejiju fang*, 60; Kajiwara Shōzen's understanding of, 60, 63–64; sources of formulas for in *Ton'ishō* and *Man'anpō*, 60
aromatic stomachics, 57–58
Avatamsaka Sutra, 62

baths: Chinese, 145 n. 14; for infants, 43; medicinal, 19, 71, 72, 145 n. 14; and *rai* treatment, 71, 72, 73
battle service reports, 91, 92, 151 n. 15; wounds noted in, 151 n. 17–18, 152 n. 19, 152 n. 21–22, 153 n. 23
Beiji jiu fang, 33
Beiji qianjin yaofang, 30, 85
Bencaojing, 50
Bian Que (Chinese physician), 74, 78, 126 n. 26, 145 n. 30
Buddhism: analogy for explaining illness of the mind, 61–62; idea of karmic illness, 68, 70, 77–83; injunction to heal, 12, 15–16, 62; nosology of illness, 77–79
Buddhist medicine: Healing Bodhisattva, 93; Healing Buddha, 74, 146 n. 31; nosology and etiology, 68–69, 70, 76, 77–81, 82–83; prayer used in, 73–74, 145 n. 30, 146 n. 31
Buddhist monks: charitable works, 15–16, 18–20; as cultural transmitters, 7–9, 10–12, 13–14, 17–18, 23; interest in medicines, 8–14, 19–20, 100–101, 126 n. 26; networks of, xiv, 7–8, 12–20, 100–101
Buddhist monks, individual: Cihong, 23; Daishi *seng*, 23; Daoguang, xix, 23; Daomiao, 23; Dōshō, 13–14, 126 n. 24; Eisai, 8–10, 110; Eison, 16, 18; Enni Ben'en, 10–14; Ennin, 7; Gahō, 81–82; Ikkyū, 60, 141 n. 63, 144 n. 6; Ippen, 15; Jisshō, 13, 14; Jōjin, 7; Jōshun, 18, 19; Kajiwara Shōzen, qv.; Kakujō, 101; Ken'i, 47; Kōshū, 81–82; Langyuan *fang*, 23; Lanxi Daolong, 17, 23; Mingji Chujun, 14; Myōnin, 24; Nichiren, 68, 78, 80, 88, 147 n. 50; Ninshō, 16, 18–19, 129 n. 47; Qingzhuo ōshō, 23; Renki, 26, 50, 138 n. 18; Rennyo, 146 n. 37
Bureau for Emending Medical Texts, 29

Changxin, 23
Chao Yuanfang, 61

Chen Shiwen, 11
Chen Yan, 61
Chen Ziming, 33, 34–35
China goods, 22, 48, 71
China ships, 22, 48
Chinese medicine: changes in, 56–57; changes in materia medica used in, 57–59; ideas on women's medicine, 41–43, 44–45; impact of printing on, 28–31; influence on Japanese wound medicine, 102–104, 104–105, 110–111; Islamic influences on, 57–59; knowledge of in Japan, 8–10, 13–14, 23, 26–27, 31–34, 37, 39–41, 42–45, 50–51, 61–62, 82–84, 85–87, 102–104; nosology and etiology, 59–60, 61, 63, 68–69, 77–79, 82–86, 87, 102–103
Chinese residents: Hakata, 6–7, 10; Kamakura, 22–23, 64; Nara, 94
Chōboji, 13, 18; and Ritsu Precept sect, 18
Chōsei ryōyōhō, 26, 50
Chu Yushi, 37, 39, 40, 134 n. 31, 135 n. 40
Cihong, 23
corpse-transmitted disease, 54, 72, 81–82, 83, 88, 118–119, 148 n. 54

Daguan bencao, 27, 52, 132 n. 4
Daidō ruijūhō, 26
Daihatsu nehan gyō. See *Mahayana Perfection of Wisdom Sutra*
Daishi *seng*, 23
Daoguang, xix, 23
Daomiao, 23
Dayiju fang, 37
Dazaifu, 4–5, 6, 10, 21
Denshibyō nijūgo hō, 81–82
Dōshō, 13–14, 126 n. 24
Dried Infant, 93–94, 154 n. 37

Eisai, 8–10, 110; and *Kissa yōjōki*, 8–10
Eisei hiyōshō, 27
Eison, 16, 18
Enni Ben'en: and China, 10; and Dōshō, 13; and Mujū Ichien, 13; in Hakata, 10; interest in medicine, 11–12, 13; support network of, 10; and Tōfukuji library, 10–11
Ennin, 7

Fengke jiyan mingfang, 33
formulas: adjusted for individual cases, 35–36; Buddhist monks, interest in, 9–10, 12–14, 126 n. 26; Chinese, changes in, 57–59; compared in *Ishinpō* and *Man'anpō*, 56–57; compared in *Waitai miyao fang* and *Hejiju fang*, 58–59; increased complexity of, 56–59; Islamic, 57–58; Kajiwara Shōzen comments on, 32–33, 39–41, 43, 51–52, 54–55, 62–65, 71–72, 86, 94–95, 126 n. 24, 140 n. 46; in *Kissa yōjōki*, 9; and *rai* illness, 71–72, 86–87; sources for in *Man'anpō* and *Ton'ishō*, 31–32; substitution of materia medica in, 55–56; *Ton'ishō* as a source for wound medicine formulas, 105–107
formulas, named: Agada Powder, 99; Alum Powder, 107; Amber Decoction, 55; Assisting Birth Powder, 43; Black Deity Powder, 45; Black Medicine, 99; Black Tin (Lead) Pill, 13; Cattail Powder, 55; Chebulic Myrobalan Pill, 132 n. 1; Chinese Cornbind Pill, 86;

Cinnabar Pill, 140 n. 56; Cinnabar Prime Pill, 55; Cloud Mother (Mica) Ointment, 106, 156 n. 72; Coiling Leek Powder, 63; Death Pill, 55; Divine Chinese-Angelica Ointment, 103; Divine Efficacy Chinese-Angelica Ointment, 94, 103; Divine Transcendent's Fundamental Ointment, 54; Eight Winds Powder, 71; Five Fragrance Powder, 36; Five Fragrances Infusion, 9, 99, 110; Grain Esteemed Powder, 65; Green Medicine, 99; Hempwind Oil, 71; Hundred Centered Powder, 65; Increased Damage Four Ingredient Decoction, 45; Jade Dragon Decoction, 107; Japan White Medicine, 108; Joy Medicine, 100; Long Life Medicine, 126 n. 24; Meeting the Transcendent Pill, 71, 72; Miraculous Desire Chinese-Artichoke Pill, 71; Mr. Guang's Response to Sensation Pill, 37; Musk Storax, 65; Neutralize Food Pill, 32; Nourishing Life Pill, 13; Nurturing Qi Decoction, 71; Nutmeg Powder, 65; Ox Gallstone Agada Pill, 65; Ox Gallstone Pure Heart Pill, 148 n. 53; Penetrating Chestnut Powder, 14; Penetrating Heaven Rebuilding Powder, 71; Perillia Syrup, 64; Purify the Spirit Powder, 45; Purple Frost Pill, 54; Purple Pill, 54; Purple Prime Pill, 54, 142 n. 76 ; Realgar Pill, 52; Rectify Qi Powder, 64; Red-Rooted Sage Ointment, 43; Silver Liquid Pill, 140 n. 46; Six Flavors Eight Flavors Calming Stomach Powder, 65; Six Ingredient Musk Pill, 132 n. 1; Soft-Shell Tortoise Shell Pill, 55; Spirit Sand Pill, 13; Storax Pill, 45, 51, 64, 142 n. 76; Sulfur Powder, 107; Thinking of Food Pill, 32; Transform the Poison Expel the Pus Inner Augmenting Powder, 106; Trembling Powder, 140 n. 46; Twelve-Ingredient Green Medicine, 101; Twin Purpose Gold Pill, 107; Warm White Pill, 108; Wax Tea, 47, 137 n. 10; White Medicine, 99; Yamato Sugimoto Ointment, 101; Yu Family Meeting the Transcendent Pill, 13, 14

Fukane Sukebito, 26, 53

Fukudenpō, 49, 137 n. 13

Fukutomi zōshi, 137 n. 16

Fumon-in Kyō Ron Shō So Goroku Jusho ra mokuroku, 125 n. 19

funaigai in, 102. *See also* "not inner or outer causes"

Furen daquan liangfang, 33, 34–35, 41, 51

Fuyukage, xix

Gahō, 81–82

Give-Five General, 101

gōbyō. *See* karmic illness

Go-Daigo (emperor), 151 n. 14

Gokurakuji, 17, 18, 19, 20, 24, 41, 68, 129 n. 46, 129 n. 48, 137 n. 16; map of, 19, 130 n. 51; medical facilities, 19–20, 24, 68

Go-Shirakawa (emperor), 5

Gotai miwakeshū, 81, 144 n. 9

Great Calming and Contemplation, 77–79; and Buddhist nosology of illness, 77–79

Great Teacher of Mt. Kōya, 101

gunchūjō. *See* battle service reports
Guo Tan, 12

Hakata, 1, 6–7, 8, 10, 18, 19, 21–22, 109; Chinese residents, 5, 6–7; religious institutions, 8, 10; trade port, 6–7, 21–22; Zen temples, 8, 10
Hanazono (emperor), 149 n. 64
Hangzhou, 46
Hanzhang, 23
Healing Bodhisattva Yakushi Kannon, 93
Healing Buddha, 74, 146 n. 31
Heian aristocracy: attitude to outside world, 2, 4–6; cultural capital of, 3–4, 26; intellectual perspectives, 3–4
Hejiju fang, 11, 30, 31, 33, 36–37, 44–45, 54, 57, 58–59, 63, 86, 95, 96, 107, 132 n. 5; editions of, 36–37; formulas, 57–59, 63, 155 n. 43; importance in *Man'anpō* and *Ton'ishō*, 31–32; Islamic medicine and, 59; postpartum care noted in, 43–45; source of formulas for *rai* treatment, 86; theory of "all forms of [disorders of] qi," 58, 59–60; Western-origin drugs in, 58–59, 63
hinin, 15, 16, 19
Hōjō family, 18, 21, 89; attitude to the new, 21; contact with the Ritsu Precept sect, 18; control of Kamakura, 20–21; destruction of, 89; support for Buddhism, 9, 17–19; trade activity, 18, 21–23
Hōjō Naritoki, 18
Hōjō Sadatoki, 48
Hōjō Shigetoki: and Ritsu (Precept) sect, 17–18; writings, 17, 80
Hōjō Takatoki, 23
Hōjō Tokimune, 23
Hōjō Tokiyori, 17
Hokiron, 24
Hokkekyō. See *Lotus Sutra*
Honzō iroha shō, 27, 36, 52, 53
Honzō wamyō, 26, 27, 47, 53, 54, 116; and identification of materia medica, 53–54
Hōryūji, 136 n. 4
Huangdi (Yellow Emperor), 78, 145 n. 29
Huangdi neijing suwen, 11, 30
Huiqing, 5, 6, 9
Huoren shizheng fang houji, 33, 96

Ibn-Sīnā, *Canon of Medicine*, 57, 58
Idanshō, 139 n. 26
Ikkyū, 60, 141 n. 63, 144 n. 6
Ippen, 15, 127 n. 29; charitable activity of, 15
Ippen shōnin eden, 15
Iryakushō, 27
Ishinpō, xiii, 26–27, 56–57, 94, 132 n. 4; as cultural capital, 27; formulas noted in, 56–57
Islamic medicine: xvi, 46; aromatic stomachics, 57; formulas, 58–59; influence in China, 56–59; influence in Japan, 59–65; materia medica used in, 58
Issaikyō, 18
Itō Sukechika, 101

Japanese medicine: attitudes to prescribing medicines, 42–43; Buddhist nosology and, 61–62; court physicians, 25–27; deficiencies noted by Kajiwara Shōzen, 38–41, 42–45, 139 n. 26; influence of Islamic medicine, 59–60, 63–65;

lineages and schools in, 9–14, 25–26, 100–101; practices in women's medicine, 41–45, 105–108; texts, 25–27; treatment facilities, 19–20; use of imported materia medica, 47–49, 71–72, 109–110
Jianyi fanglun, 33, 96
Jiayou buzhu bencao, 30
Jingui yaolüe fanglun, 30, 133 n. 8
Jingxiao chanbao, 134 n. 21
Jingyi fang, 39
Jingzhilu, 136 n. 2
Jisshō, 13, 14
Jisshō-in, 13
Jivaka (Indian physician), 9, 74, 78, 145 n. 29–30, 147 n. 50
Jōjin, 7
Jōshun, 18, 19
Jōtenji, 10

Kaibao xinxiang ding bencao, 29
Kajiwara Shōzen, xiii, xv, xvi, xvii, xviii, xix, xx, 2, 12–14, 20, 23–25, 27, 31–34, 36–46, 48–55, 59–68, 71–74, 76–79, 81–89, 95–96, 100, 102, 104, 106, 108, 110, 113–119; access to Chinese medical works, 31–34; access to Japanese medical works, 25–26, 50, 52; activity in Kamakura, 20, 24; engagement of formulas, 32–33, 63–65, 71–72, 86, 94; formulas of, 54–55, 64–65, 142 n. 74; and identification of materia medica, 52–55; overview of Song medicine, 34–37; understanding of "all forms of disorders of qi," 59, 61, 62–63; understanding of "not inner or outer cause," 61, 102; writings, xviii–xx
Kajiwara Shōzen, and *rai*: analyses and descriptions of, 68–71, 74–77, 84–87; different understanding of in *Ton'ishō* and *Man'anpō*, 83–87; treatments for, 70–74
Kajiwara Shōzen, comments on: failings of Japanese medicine, 38–40, 42–45, 53–54; formulas, 32–33, 39–41, 51–52, 54–55, 63–65, 71–72, 86–87, 94, 126 n. 24, 140 n. 46; illnesses, 38–39, 78–79; karmic illness, 84–87; measurements, 49–51; medical treatment for women, 41–45, 105–108; new Chinese medicinal knowledge, 38–41; qi, 40, 43, 60, 62, 63, 64, 71, 82, 87, 118, 141 n. 64, 142 n. 67
Kakujō, 101
Kamakura *bakufu*: attitude to commerce, 21–22; attitude to new knowledge, 21; control of by Hōjō family, 21–22; destruction of, 48, 89, 90; lack of wound medicine specialists, 94; openness to overseas contacts, 21–24; physicians and, 23, 24, 94; and public welfare, 16–17, 19; and Ritsu (Precept) sect, 17–19; support for Buddhism, 17–18
Kamakura city, xiv, 16–17, 20–23, 48, 89, 93, 109; commerce, 22–23, 47–48; overseas residents, 23, 64; physicians in, 14, 19, 23, 24, 64, 94; warfare in, 89
Kamakura Great Buddha, 17, 19, 22
Kanazawa Bunko library, 17–18, 24
Kanezawa Sadaaki, 22
Kanezawa Sanetoki, 17–18
karabune. *See* China ships
karamono. *See* China goods

karma, 15–16, 76–77, 77–80, 82–84, 87, 88, 118–119, 147 n. 50
karmic illness (*gōbyō*), 68, 70, 76, 77–80, 146 n. 37; and corpse transmitted disease, 81–84; disagreements concerning identification of, 81–82, 83; in *Gotai miwakeshū*, 81; Hōjō Shigetoki's understanding of, 80; Kajiwara Shōzen's changing views on, 77–78, 80; Kajiwara Shōzen's general understanding of, 82–84; in *Mahayana Perfection of Wisdom Sutra*, 79; Nichiren's views of, 77–78, 80; *rai* as a karmic illness, 16, 70, 76–77, 81; in *Sanyin fang*, 82–83
kawaramono, 15
Kawatsu Lay Priest, 101, 155 n. 53
Kazō hihō/Jiacang mifang, 11, 12
Kegon kyō. See *Avatamsaka Sutra*
Kenchōji, 17
Ken'i, 47
Kenninji, 8
Keyong fang, 33, 39, 60, 96
Khubilai Khan (emperor), 35
Kihō, 48, 89–90, 97, 98–100, 101, 104, 108, 109, 110; table of contents, 98–100
Kinsō ryōjishō, 48, 90, 97–98, 100, 101, 102, 103, 104, 108, 110; table of contents, 97–98
Kissa yōjōki, 8–10, 110; indicative of new engagement with China, 9–10; materia medica in, 9
Kōjishō, 47
Koremune Tomotoshi, 27, 36, 57
Kōshū, 81–82
Kōyakushō, 47
Kōyōshō, 47
Kujō Michiie, 10, 11
Langyuan *fang*, 23
Lanxi Daolong, 17, 23
leprosy. See *rai*
Li Minshou, 33
Lotus Sutra, 78, 79, 147 n. 45; on karma and body condition, 79

Mahāparinirvāna Sutra. See *Mahayana Perfection of Wisdom Sutra*
Mahayana Perfection of Wisdom Sutra, 79
Maka shikan. See *Great Calming and Contemplation*
Man'anpō, xiii, xvii, xix–xx, 12, 23, 31, 32, 33, 35, 37, 41, 42, 49, 52, 55, 56, 57–58, 59, 60, 63, 68, 72, 83, 84–87, 95–96, 102, 115; Chinese medical works used in, 31–34; contents, xix–xx; corpse-transmitted disease in, 83–84; discussion of *rai*, 84–87; discussion of *rai* contrasted to discussion of in *Ton'ishō*, 85–87; Long Life Medicine praised in, 126 n. 24; measuring standards noted in, 50–52, 138 n. 19, 138 n. 21, 139 n. 40; sources of formulas in, 31–32, 59–60; Storax Pill praised in, 64; women's medicine noted in, 41–45; wound medicine in, 95–96
Mañjuśrī Bodhisattva, xv, 12, 14, 15, 16, 127 n. 30
materia medica: availability, 47–49, 55–56, 109, 140 n. 46, 140 n. 50; in Chinese formulas, 57–59, 140 n. 57; Chinese origins of, 58, 63, 140 n. 57, 142 n. 78, 143 n. 79; in *Hejiju fang*, 57–59; identification of, 52–54, 139 n. 26, 139 n. 43; in Islamic formulas, 57–58; measurement standards for, 50–52,

138 n. 18–19, 138 n. 21, 138 n. 25, 139 n. 40; in *Shenghui fang*, 58–59; Southeast Asian origins of, 49, 136 n. 2; specific items of, 9, 32, 37, 40, 43, 47–49, 50–51, 53–57, 58, 59, 64, 65, 93, 108, 109, 110, 134 n. 27, 136 n. 2, 136 n. 4, 137 n. 10, 137 n. 12, 137 n. 16, 138 n. 19, 139 n. 43, 140 n. 57, 141 n. 60, 142 n. 69, 142 n. 78, 143 n. 79, 157 n. 89; substitution of, 55–56; terminology, 54–55; trade in, 46–49, 136 n. 2; types used in wound medicine, 93–94, 109–110; in *Waitai miyao fang*, 58–59; Western origins of, 58–59, 63–65, 141 n. 59–60, 142 n. 78

measurement standards and materia medica, 50–52, 138 n. 18–19, 138 n. 21, 138 n. 25, 139 n. 40

medical figures, legendary: Bian Que (Chinese physician), 74, 79, 126 n. 26, 145 n. 29; Huangdi (Yellow Emperor), 78, 145 n. 29; Jivaka (Indian physician), 9, 74, 78, 145 n. 29–30, 147 n. 50; Shennong, 8, 78; Yu Fu (Chinese physician), 126 n. 26

medical works, Chinese: 9, 10–12, 27; alternative theories of *rai*, 85–87; availability of in Japan, 9, 10–12, 26–27, 31ff., 52; influence on wound medicine, 95–96, 102–103, 111; Northern Song, 29–30; Song print revolution and, 28–30; Southern Song, 30; titles utilized in *Man'anpō* and *Ton'ishō*, 30–37

medical works, Chinese, specific titles: *Beiji jiu fang*, 33; *Beiji qianjin yaofang*, 30, 85; *Bencaojing*, 50; *Daguan bencao*, 27, 52, 132 n. 4; *Dayiju fang*, 37; *Fengke jiyan mingfang*, 33; *Furen daquan liangfang*, 33, 34–35, 41, 51; *Hejiju fang*, 11, 30, 31, 33, 36–37, 44–45, 54, 57, 58–59, 63, 86, 95, 96, 107, 132 n. 5; *Huangdi neijing suwen*, 11, 30; *Huoren shizheng fang houji*, 33, 96; *Jianyi fanglun*, 33, 96; *Jiayou buzhu bencao*, 30; *Jingui yaolüe fanglun*, 30, 133 n. 8; *Jingxiao chanbao*, 134 n. 21; *Jingyi fang*, 39; *Kaibao xinxiang ding bencao*, 29; *Kazō hihō/Jiacang mifang*, 11, 12; *Keyong fang*, 33, 39, 60, 96; *Puji benshi fang*, 12, 33, 36, 95; *Qianjin fang*, 31, 43, 44, 57, 102; *Rencun Sunshi zhibing huofa mifang*, 33, 83–84, 118; *Sanyin fang*, 31, 43, 51, 60, 61, 63, 82, 85, 86, 87, 102, 103, 104, 107, 111, 118; *Shanghan huorenshu*, 11; *Shanghan lun*, 30, 57, 133 n. 11; *Shenghui fang*, 30, 31, 43, 44, 58, 59, 82, 85; *Shengji fang*, 96; *Shengji zonglu*, 32, 39, 59, 60, 64, 85, 86, 87; *Shibian liangfang*, 12; *Shizhai baiyi xuanfang*, 33, 95; *Suwen jing*, 11; *Tong Zhenzi maijue*, 11; *Waike jingyao*, 33; *Waitai miyao fang*, 43, 44, 58–59, 140 n. 57; *Wang Shuhe maijue*, 11; *Wanquan fang*, 140 n. 46; *Weishi jiacang fang*, 12, 33, 34, 141 n. 60; *Xu yijian fang*, 33; *Yangsheng biyong fang*, 37, 39–40, 139 n. 31; *Yangshi jiacang fang*, 33, 34; *Yanshi jisheng fang*, 33, 82; *Yeshi luyan fang*, 33, 104; *Yifan jicheng*, 133 n. 19; *Yijian fang*, 12, 33; *Yishuo*, 33; *Youyou xinshu*, 32,

37, 51, 56, 140 n. 46; *Yuyaoyuan fang*, 32, 33, 35, 60, 96, 155 n. 49; *Zatsuzatsu hō/Zaza fang*, 11, 12; *Zhenzhong fang*, 11; *Zhubing yuanhou zonglun*, 61
medical works, Japanese: 25–27; dearth of, 25–27; deficiencies of, 27, 38–41, 50; as response to social need, 67–68, 74, 88–89, 100–103
medical works, Japanese, specific titles: *Chōsei ryōyōhō*, 26, 50; *Daidō ruijūhō*, 26; *Denshibyō nijūgo hō*, 81–82; *Eisei hiyōshō*, 27; *Fukudenpō*, 49, 137 n. 13; *Gotai miwakeshū*, 81, 144 n. 9; *Hokiron*, 24; *Honzō iroha shō*, 27, 36, 52, 53; *Honzō wamyō*, 26, 27, 47, 53, 54, 116; *Idanshō*, 139 n. 26; *Iryakushō*, 27; *Ishinpō*, xiii, 26–27, 56–57, 94; *Kazō hihō/ Jiacang mifang*, 11, 12; *Kihō*, 48, 89–90, 97, 98–100, 101, 104, 108, 109, 110; *Kinsō ryōjishō*, 48, 90, 97–98, 100, 101, 102, 103, 104, 108, 110; *Kissa yōjōki*, 8–10, 110; *Kōjishō*, 47; *Kōyakushō*, 47; *Kōyōshō*, 47; *Man'anpō*, xiii, xvii, xix–xx, 12, 23, 31, 32, 33, 35, 37, 41, 42, 49, 52, 55, 56, 57–58, 60, 63, 68, 72, 83, 84–87, 95–96, 102, 115; *Shōchūhō*, 132 n. 4; *Shōmi kagami*, 52, 53, 139 n. 27; *Ton'ishō*, xiii, xvii, xviii, xix, xx, 24, 26, 31, 37, 38, 41, 42–43, 49, 52, 54, 59, 60, 68, 70, 73, 74, 81, 84, 85, 86, 87, 95, 100, 104, 105, 106, 115; *Yakumei ruijū*, 52–53; *Yakushō*, 11; *Yakushushō*, 47; *Yōketsushō*, 11; *Zatsuzatsu hō/Zaza fang*, 11, 12
medical writers, Buddhist monks: Eisai, 8–10, 110; Gahō, 81–82; Kajiwara Shōzen, qv.; Ken'i, 47; Kōshū, 81–82; Renki, 26, 50, 138 n. 18; Zhiyi, 77–79
medical writers, Chinese: Chao Yuanfang, 61; Chen Shiwen, 11; Chen Yan, 61; Chen Ziming, 33, 34–35; Chu Yushi, 37, 39, 40, 134 n. 31, 135 n. 40; Guo Tan, 12; Li Minshou, 33; Sun Rencun, 83, 84, 112; Sun Simiao, 11, 20, 41, 85, 135 n. 43; Sun Yunxian, 133 n. 19; Wang Huaiyin, 85; Wang Shuhe, 11; Wang Shuo, 12; Wei Xian, 12, 34; Xu Guozhen, 33, 35; Xu Shuwei, 12, 36; Yang Tan, 34; Zan Yin, 134 n. 21; Zhang Zhongjing, 30, 133 n. 8; Zhiyi, 77–79; Zhu Gong, 11
medical writers, Japanese: Eisai, 8–10, 11; Fukane Sukebito, 26, 53; Gahō, 81–82; Kajiwara Shōzen, qv.; Ken'i, 47; Koremune Tomotoshi, 27, 36, 57; Kōshū, 81–82; Renki, 26, 50, 138 n. 18; Tanba Masatada, 27; Tanba Yasuyori, 26; Tanba Yukinaga, 27; Tominokōji Norizane, 89–90, 150 n. 3; Wake Tadakage, 48
Minamoto Sanetomo, 9
Mingji Chujun, 14
Mingtangtu, 11
Mingtangtu jing, 11
Mingzhou, 46
Mohe ziguan. See *Great Calming and Contemplation*
Mongol invasions of Japan, 10, 48, 90
Mountain Ailment, 69, 70, 71, 73, 75–76, 84, 108. See also *rai*
Mujū Ichien, 13–14, 18; medical interests of, 13

Munakata Shrine, 6, 10; Chinese women and, 6–7
Myōan Eisai. *See* Eisai
Myōnin (head of Shōmyōji), 24

Nagai Munehide, 24
Nagai Sadahide, 23
Nanfu Lay Priest, 101, 156 n. 61
New Administrative Regulations of 1261, 17, 128 n. 38
Nichiren, 68, 78, 80–81, 88; view of karmic illness, 78, 80–81; views on illness, 78, 147 n. 50; views on karma, 147 n. 50
Nikaidō bureaucrat family, 22
Nikaidō Yukifuji, 24, 131 n. 66
Ningbo, 1, 6, 46
Ninshō, 16, 18–19, 130 n. 49; and Gokurakuji temple, 18–19; and Hōjō family, 18; public welfare activity, 18–19; ten vows of, 129 n. 47
"not inner or outer causes": mentioned by Kajiwara Shōzen, nosology articulated in *Sanyin fang*, 102; theoretical basis for wound medicine, 102–104, 111
not-eating illness, 9, 40

overseas contacts, Japanese attitudes to, 3–7, 8–10, 21–23

permitted and prohibited foods, 53, 72–73, 94–95, 139 n. 26
physicians and pharmacists: in Kamakura, 14, 19, 23, 24, 64, 94; in Kyoto, 12, 13, 26–27, 48, 94; in Kyushu, 5, 6, 9, 125 n. 17; in Nara, 94
physicians and pharmacists (non-authors), Chinese: Geng Langzhong, 126 n. 26; Hanzhang, 23; Huiqing, 5, 6, 9; Langyuan *fang*, 23; Zhiguang, 64
physicians and pharmacists (non-authors), Japanese: Daizenbō, 125 n. 17; Dōshō, 13–14, 126 n. 24; Give-Five General, 101; Great Teacher of Mt. Kōya, 101; Itō Sukechika, 101; Kakujō, 101; Kawatsu Lay Priest, 101, 155 n. 53; Kenshōbō, 125 n. 17; Nanfu Lay Priest, 101, 156 n. 61; Rakuami (wound physician), 155 n. 50; Shichirō "Boat-Captain" Funagashira, 101; Tōtōmi Lay Priest, 101; Uritsu no kan, 101; Wake Tadakage, 48
printing: and medical publication in Song, 29–30; printed medical works and Kajiwara Shōzen, 31–37; Song revolution in, 28–29
Puji benshi fang, 12, 33, 36, 95

qi, 40, 44, 46, 59–60, 62, 63, 64, 71, 75, 82, 87, 141 n. 64, 142 n. 67, 143 n. 56; disorders of, 57, 58, 59–62, 63, 64, 102; of infants, 43; Kajiwara Shōzen's comments on, 60, 62, 141 n. 64, 142 n. 67; of postpartum women, 44; relation to the prescribing of medicines, 40–41. *See also* "all forms of [disorders of] qi"
Qianjin fang, 31, 43, 44, 57, 102
Qingzhuo ōshō, 23

rai: Buddhist views of, 15–16, 68–70, 76–77; Chinese views of, 84–87; determination of symptoms as, 67–68, 68–70, 144 n. 9; Japanese colloquial terms for, 68, 74–77

(*see also* Mountain Ailment); Kajiwara Shōzen's views of, 68–71, 74–77, 84–87; as a karmic illness, 16, 70, 76–77; mantra used in treatment, 73–74; medicines for, 71–72, 86–87; patient numbers, 19–20, 130 n. 53; social attitudes toward, 67–68, 143 n. 5, 144 n. 6; treatment facilities, 19–20; treatment prohibitions, 72–73; treatment taboos, 73, 156 n. 70; treatments for, 70–74, 86; understanding of in *Man'anpō*, 84–87; understanding of in *Ton'ishō*, 68–71, 74–77, 84–87; variant names for, 69, 74–77, 85–86; varieties of, 74–77, 85–86
Rakuami (wound physician), 155 n. 50
Rencun Sunshi zhibing huofa mifang, 33, 83–84, 118
Renki, 26, 50, 138 n. 18
Rennyo, 146 n. 37
Ritsu Precept sect, xiv–xv, 1, 2, 14, 15–16, 18, 19; welfare activity in Kamakura, 18–20

Saddharma Puṇḍarīka Sutra. See *Lotus Sutra*
Saidaiji, 26
Sanyin fang, 31, 43, 51, 60, 61, 63, 82, 85, 86, 87, 102, 103, 104, 107, 111, 118; influence on wound medicine, 102–104; information on *rai*, 84–85, 87; nosology of illness, 60–61; as source in *Ton'ishō* and *Man'anpō*, 31; theory of "not inner or outer causes," 102–103; views on qi, 61, 63, 141 n. 64
Sekiso ōrai, 137 n. 12
Shanghan huorenshu, 11
Shanghan lun, 30, 57, 133 n. 11
Shasekishū, 13
Shenghui fang, 30, 31, 43, 44, 58, 59, 82, 85
Shengji fang, 96
Shengji zonglu, 32, 39, 59, 60, 64, 85, 86, 87; major source for *Man'anpō*, 32; source for wound medicine in *Man'anpō*, 95–96, 102; views on *rai* cited, 85, 87
Shennong, 8, 78
Shibian liangfang, 12
Shichirō "Boat-Captain" Funagashira, 101
Shingon, 25, 26
Shinsarugaku ki, 47, 48
Shizhai baiyi xuanfang, 33, 95
Shōchūhō, 132 n. 4
Shōfukuji, 8
Shōmi kagami, 52, 53, 139 n. 27
Shōmyōji, 18, 23, 24
Shōni Sukeyoshi, 10
Shōzen. *See* Kajiwara Shōzen
Storax Pill, 45, 51, 64, 65, 142 n. 69
Su (Chinese boat captain), 6
Sun Rencun, 83, 84
Sun Simiao, 11, 30, 41, 85, 135 n. 43
Sun Yunxian, 133 n. 19
Suwen jing, 11

Taiping huimin Hejiju fang. See *Hejiju fang*
Taiping Shenghui fang. See *Shenghui fang*
Taiping yulan, 4, 9–10, 28
Taira Kiyomori, 5
Tanba family, 26, 27, 132 n. 2, 132 n. 4, 137 n. 12
Tanba Masatada, 27
Tanba Yasuyori, 26
Tanba Yukinaga, 27

tea: availability in Kamakura, 22, 48; in *Kissa yōjōki*, 8–9; as materia medica, 8–9, 48, 137 n. 10
Tendai, 25, 26
Tōdaiji, 17
Tōfukuji, 10–13, 34; medical activity at, 12–13; medical books in library of, 10–12, 34
Tominokōji Norizane, 89–90, 150 n. 3
Tong Zhenzi maijue, 11
Ton'ishō, xiii, xvii, xviii, xix, xx, 24, 26, 31, 37, 38, 41, 42–43, 49, 52, 54, 59, 60, 68, 70, 73, 74, 81, 84, 85, 86, 87, 95, 100, 104, 105, 106, 115; Chinese medical works used in, 31, 59; circulated in Kamakura, 24; contents, xix; corpse-transmitted disease, 83; discussion of qi, 60–62, 141 n. 64, 142 n. 67; information on women's medicine, 105–108; karma noted in, 81, 87; karmic illness in, 81–83; mantras used in, 74, 145 n. 30; nosology of disease in, 60–62, 78–79; prohibited foods noted in, 73; purpose of compilation, xiii, xviii, 104; as source of information for wound medicine, 105–108; sources of formulas, 31, 59–60, 85–86
Ton'ishō, *rai* addressed in: categories of, 74–77; contrasted to discussion of in *Man'anpō*, 84–87; description of, 68–70, 75–77; formulas for noted in, 71–72; karmic varieties of, 76–77; treatment of, 70–74
Tōtōmi Lay Priest, 101
trade: ceramics, 22; Kamakura and, 21–22, 109, 129 n. 48; Kyushu and, 4–5, 6–7, 10, 109; luxury goods, 22–23; materia medica, 46–49, 55–56, 109–110, 136 n. 2
Tripitaka, 28
Tsūken nyūdō zōsho mokuroku, 132 n. 4

Uritsu no kan, 101

Vimalakirti, 145 n. 29–30

Waike jingyao, 33
Waitai miyao fang, 43, 44, 58–59, 140 n. 57; materia medica in, 58–59
Wakaejima port, 21
Wake family, 26
Wake Tadakage, 48
Wang, Ms. (Chinese woman in Hakata), 6–7, 125 n. 12
Wang Huaiyin, 85
Wang Shuhe, 11
Wang Shuhe maijue, 11
Wang Shuo, 12
Wanquan fang, 140 n. 46
Wanshou Chansi, 10
warfare, Japanese: before 1330s, 92–96; casualties in, 92; changes in, 90–92; numbers engaged in, 153 n. 25, 153 n. 27; weapons, 91, 104, 151 n. 15, 152 n. 20; wounds incurred, 91–92, 109–110, 152 n. 20
Wei Xian, 12, 34
Weishi jiacang fang, 12, 33, 34, 141 n. 60
women's medicine: deficiencies in Japan, 42–43, 44; Kajiwara Shōzen's comments on, 41–45; as major medical topic, 41–42; menstruation, 35, 42, 55, 107; menstruation, taboos and, 73, 106; morning sickness, 42, 43;

new Chinese knowledge regarding, 34–35, 42–45; postpartum care, 44–45, 106–108; pregnancy and birth, 42–45, 95, 106–108; 135 n. 50; as source for wound medicine, 105–108, 156 n. 68; suppositories, 107; umbilical cords, 43, 110, 136 n. 53
wound medicine: application to women's medicine, 108; Chinese influence on, 101–105, 110–111; emergence as a specialty, 89–91, 110–111; injuries 94–96, 96–100, 101, 104, 150 n. 11, 151 n. 16–18, 152 n. 19–21, 152 n. 22, 153 n. 23, 153 n. 29, 154 n. 31; and *Ishinpō*, 94; and *Man'anpō*, 95–96; materia medica used in, 93–94, 109–110, 154 n. 37; medicines, 101, 103, 108, 110; prior to 1330s, 92–96; and *Sanyin fang*, 102–104; sources of knowledge for, 93–94, 94–96, 100–105, 105–108; specialists, 93–94, 100–101; texts, 89–90; texts, *Kihō*, 90, 97–98, 108; texts, *Kinsō ryōjishō*, 89, 98–99, 108; theoretical basis of, 102–104, 111; and *Ton'ishō*, 94–95; *Ton'ishō* as a source for, 105–107; treatment, taboos, and avoidances, 95, 106; treatments, 92–94, 101–102, 109, 153 n. 27; women's medicine as a source for, 105–108
wounds, 90–93, 96, 97–99, 102–103, 151 n. 17–18, 152 n. 19–22, 153 n. 23, 153 n. 29–30, 154 n. 31

Xie Guoming (Hakata Chinese merchant), 10, 125 n. 18
Xu Guozhen, 33, 35
Xu Shuwei, 12, 36
Xu yijian fang, 33

Yakumei ruijū, 52–53
Yakushō, 11
Yakushushō, 47
Yamai no sōshi, 94, 154 n. 39
Yang Rong, 6
Yang Tan, 34
Yangsheng biyong fang, 37, 39–40, 134 n. 31
Yangshi jiacang fang, 33, 34
Yanshi jisheng fang, 33, 82
Yeshi luyan fang, 33, 104
Yi, Presider (Kamakura bakufu agent), 22–23
Yifan jicheng, 133 n. 19
Yijian fang, 12, 33
Yishuo, 33
Yōketsushō, 11
Youyou xinshu, 32, 37, 51, 56, 140 n. 46
Yu Fu (Chinese physician), 126 n. 26
Yueguang, and mistaken perception, 62
Yuyaoyuan fang, 32, 33, 35, 60, 96, 155 n. 49

Zan Yin, 134 n. 21
Zatsuzatsu hō/*Zaza fang*, 11, 12
Zhang, Ms. (Chinese woman in Hakata), 6–7, 125 n. 12
Zhang Guang'an, 6
Zhang Zhongjing, 30, 133 n. 8
Zhenzhong fang, 11
Zhiguang, 64
Zhiyi, 77–79
Zhu Gong, 11
Zhubing yuanhou zonglun, 61

ABOUT THE AUTHOR

A specialist on medieval Japan, Andrew Edmund Goble's interdisciplinary research spans a wide range of topics. His earlier publications included such topics as the Kamakura warrior government, social and political change and the fourteenth-century Kenmu revolution, and the intellectual profile of Emperor Hanazono. His recent research has focused on premodern and medical history. In addition to topics taken up in the present work, his latest publications include "Images of Illness: Interpreting the Medieval *Scrolls of Afflictions*" (in *Currents in Medieval Japanese History*), and "Rhythms of Medicine and Community in Late Sixteenth Century Japan: Yamashina Tokitsune (1543–1611) and His Patients" (in *East Asian Science, Technology, and Medicine*, No. 29, 2008). He is recently coeditor of *Tools of Culture: Japan's Cultural, Intellectual, Medical, and Technological Contacts in East Asia, 1000s–1500s* (2009), and *Currents in Medieval Japanese History: Essays in Honor of Jeffrey P. Mass* (2009). Professor Goble teaches at the University of Oregon.

Production Notes for Goble | *Confluences of Medicine in Medieval Japan*

Cover design by Julie Matsuo-Chun

Text design and composition by Jansom
with display type in Bodega Sans
and text type in Adobe Garamond Pro

Printing and binding by Sheridan Books, Inc.

Printed on 55 lb. House Natural, 360 ppi